医学英語
Communication & Writing
能力アップ！

著　土居 治・西村 真澄・David Chart
イラスト　茨木 保

金芳堂

はじめに

　最近，外国からの患者さんを診察する機会が増え，また国際会議や留学など英語でのコミュニケーションの必要性が高まっています．一方，「英語の論文は読めるが，話すことや書くことはちょっと苦手で，英語は自信がありません．」との先生方の声が多く聞かれます．実際は，会話の流れによって様々な表現方法があり，自然な英語表現を身につけるには相当な時間を要するかと思われます．そこで，本書は，「英語で意思疎通を図ることは，そんなに難しいことではない」ということをお伝えし，すぐに臨床の場面で英会話を始めて頂けるよう工夫しました．

　さて，米国テキスト「USMLE step2 CS：Tips for Being Understood by Your SP」，「Writing, Speaking, Communication Skills for Health Professionals」などでも，まず，患者さんとのコミュニケーションを取る上で「短い文で，平易な単語を使うこと」が大変重要であると指摘しています．本書は，実践の会話に役立つよう，頻繁に用いられかつ幅広く応用できる短文例をパターン化しました．また，練習問題では，パターン文例を応用することで，さらに会話を広げられるよう工夫しました．

　最後に，本書ならびにCDを繰り返しチェックして頂きました4名の英国，米国の先生方（レジデント他），また本書を出版する機会を与えて戴いた金芳堂編集長宇山閑文氏はじめ編集部各位に深謝いたします．

—— One of the best ways to improve your English speaking is not to translate Japanese literally but to imitate native speakers speaking ——

2012年2月

土居　治
西村真澄

はじめに

To help busy doctors and medical personnel to get to that stage as quickly as possible, this book introduces simple sentence patterns that can be used very widely. There are, of course, many ways to say these things in English, but short and simple sentences are the best when the most important thing is being clear.

If, once you have mastered these patterns, you want to improve the level and flexibility of your English, then it is our hope that this book will serve as a useful foundation. If, on the other hand, you only have time to learn the English necessary to make yourself understood, we hope that this book will enable you to do so as quickly as possible.

David Chart

著者・症例執筆者紹介　Profile

著

土居　治（どい　おさむ）
医学博士．どいこどもクリニック院長．山口大学医学部卒．
略歴：国立岡山病院小児医療センター小児科／小児外科，国立呉病院母子医療センター小児外科，Royal Children's Hospital, Melbourne（学位論文発表），木山病院副院長．
著書：Research Methods, Edited by Ben Greenstein, Harwood Academic Publishers.
趣味：バドミントン，ウォーキング，ガーデニング（クリニックの花が咲くのが楽しみ）．
モットー：温故知新（医療も含め日進月歩する世界には，古くからの教訓が生きている）．

著・翻訳

西村真澄（にしむら　ますみ）
薬剤師・医療通訳・医療翻訳．京都薬科大学卒．
略歴：モントレ国際大学院翻訳科 1 年終了後，ニューヨークにて医学英語を学ぶ．三菱ウエルファーマー・日本医薬情報センター海外文献部翻訳，AIT センターで医療通訳，医療翻訳・医学部予備校英語講師・東京女子医大薬剤部．
著書：赤本シリーズ「私立医大の英語」（教学社），「合格する医歯薬への英語」（東京コア），「医系英語の速読記述特訓」（東京コア）．
趣味：エアロビクス，旅行．

翻訳

David Chart（ディヴィッド・チャート）
ライター，エディター．ケンブリッジ大学卒・ケンブリッジ大学院卒．
略歴：元ケンブリッジ大学講師・日本語検定一級．
著書：「A Theory of Understanding」（Ashgate），「Heirs to Merlin」（Atlas Games），「Akrasia: Thief of Time」（Eden Studios），「Power and Privilege」（Eden Studios），「Splintered Peace」（Atlas Games），「Love and War」（Atlas Games），「The Medieval Players' Guide」（Green Ronin），「Spires of Altdorf」（Black Industries），「Knights of the Grail」（Black Industries），「Renegade Crowns」（Black Industries），「Ars Magica」Fifth Edition（Atlas Games），他．
趣味：読書，ウォーキング，旅行．
モットー：明らかなことは何もない．

カバー・本文イラスト

茨木　保（いばらき　たもつ）
医学博士．いばらきレディースクリニック院長．奈良県立医科大学卒．
略歴：大和成和病院婦人科部長．
著書：「まんが医学の歴史」（医学書院），「がんばれ！猫山先生」（日本医事新報社），「患者さんゴメンナサイ」（PHP 研究所），「医師という生き方」（発見！しごと偉人伝）（ぺりかん社）他．
趣味：猫と遊ぶ．
モットー：暗いと不平を言うよりも，すすんで明かりをつけましょう．

症例執筆

内　科

荒木康史（あらき　やすし）

医学博士．はるひ野内科クリニック院長．日本大学医学部卒．
略歴：大分市アルメイダ病院内科，日本大学医学部第2内科（現循環器内科），春日部市立病院内科，相模原協同病院循環器科医長，東十条病院循環器科部長．
趣味：音楽（ヴァイオリン演奏，医科記念オーケストラコンサートマスター）．
モットー：患者さんが元気で快適な生活を送れるよう，助力すること．

大村素子（おおむら　もとこ）

大村内科循環器科クリニック院長．奈良県立医科大学卒．
略歴：国立呉病院内科，川崎病院内科，兵庫県立西宮病院循環器内科．
趣味：旅行，民俗学．
モットー：一期一会．

小児科

土居　治

産婦人科

茨木　保

整形外科

替地恭介（かえち　きょうすけ）

医学博士．はるひ野整形外科院長．宮崎医科大学卒．
略歴：津久井赤十字病院整形外科部長．
趣味：読書．

皮膚科

段野貴一郎（だんの　きいちろう）

医学博士．だんの皮フ科クリニック院長．京都大学卒．
著書：「ここがツボ　患者に伝える皮膚外用剤の使い方」（金芳堂），「皮膚疾患最新の治療2009-2010」（分担）（南江堂），「透析室に置きたいかゆみ治療パーフェクトガイド」（金芳堂）．
略歴：滋賀医科大学皮膚科准教授．
趣味：写真，書画研究．

眼　科

土井治道（どい　はるみち）

医学博士．土井眼科院長．関西医科大学卒．
略歴：関西医科大学眼科，大阪市立住吉市民病院眼科医長．
趣味：播磨古代史探究．

歯　科

辻本　美穂（つじもと　みほ）

博士．東京医科歯科大学歯科医師．日本大学歯学部卒．東京医科歯科大学大学院卒．
略歴：虎の門病院歯科．

本書の使い方

A　本書の読み方

Part 1　Communication 編
1. まず「パターン」を確認します．時間があれば「このパターンでこれだけ話せる！」で確認しましょう．
2. 次に，症例部分を読みます．

Part 2　Basic Medical Writing 編
　　短時間で「基本的な writing」の練習ができるように工夫しています．

B　CD の聴き方

1. 各科ごとに最初に「パターン」が流れます．これは，本文の「パターン」を CD 用に再構成した内容です．
2. 次に，目次に（英・日）印がついた「Case」が，英語と日本語で流れます．
3. 最後に，目次に（英・日）および（英）印がついた「Case」の英会話が流れます．聞こえなかった音の単語を出来る限り本で確認し，繰り返しお聞きください．

《listening 力をつけるコツ》
　　'r' 'l' 'f' 'b' 'th' 'p' などの日本語にない音を繰り返し聞いて身につけます．単音が聞こえ出すと，全体文がどんどん聞こえてきます．また，「強弱強弱強弱弱」といった「塊のイントネーション」に乗せて聞くように心がけましょう．
　　CD では，コントラクション（45 頁参照）を多く用いています．数語または短文を「一語」のように聞きなれて，シャドウイング（英語を追いかけて口に出す）をしながら実用表現を増やしましょう．

CD 目次　CD Index

CD 1		トラック番号	
内　科		1	パターン
	(英語・日本語)	2	ケース 1-1, 1-2　34 歳女性
	(英語・日本語)	3	ケース 2-1　54 歳男性
	(英語・日本語)	4	ケース 3　45 歳男性
	(英語・日本語)	5	ケース 5　66 歳女性
	(英語)	6	CASE1-1, 1-2　34-year-old woman
	(英語)	7	CASE2-1　54-year-old man
	(英語)	8	CASE3　45-year-old man
	(英語)	9	CASE4-1, 4-2　26-year-old woman
	(英語)	10	CASE5　66-year-old woman
小児科		11	パターン
	(英語・日本語)	12	ケース 6-1, 6-2　母親が生後 11 ヵ月男児を連れて受診
	(英語・日本語)	13	ケース 7-1　母親が 7 歳女児を連れて受診
	(英語・日本語)	14	ケース 9-1　母親が生後 10 ヵ月男児を連れ，健診のため来院
	(英語・日本語)	15	ケース 10-1　母親が 5 歳男児を連れて受診
	(英語)	16	CASE6-1, 6-2　11-month-old boy
	(英語)	17	CASE7-1, 7-2　7-year-old girl
	(英語)	18	CASE8-1, 8-2　5-month-old boy
	(英語)	19	CASE9-1　10-month-old boy
	(英語)	20	CASE10-1　5-year-old boy

CD 2		トラック番号	
産婦人科		1	パターン
	(英語・日本語)	2	ケース 12-1, 12-2　34 歳女性
	(英語・日本語)	3	ケース 13　41 歳女性
	(英語)	4	CASE11-1, 11-2　26-year-old woman
	(英語)	5	CASE12-1, 12-2, 12-3　34-year-old woman
	(英語)	6	CASE13　41-year-old woman
整形外科		7	パターン
	(英語・日本語)	8	ケース 14　20 歳男性
	(英語・日本語)	9	ケース 15-1　32 歳男性
	(英語・日本語)	10	ケース 16-1　75 歳女性
	(英語・日本語)	11	ケース 17　24 歳女性
	(英語)	12	CASE14　20-year-old man
	(英語)	13	CASE15-1, 15-2　32-year-old man
	(英語)	14	CASE16-1, 16-2　75-year-old woman
	(英語)	15	CASE17　24-year-old woman
皮膚科		16	パターン
	(英語・日本語)	17	ケース 18-1, 18-2　50 歳男性
	(英語・日本語)	18	ケース 19-1　22 歳女性
	(英語)	19	CASE18-1, 18-2　50-year-old woman
	(英語)	20	CASE19-1, 19-2　22-year-old woman
眼科		21	パターン
	(英語・日本語)	22	ケース 22　30 歳女性
	(英語・日本語)	23	ケース 23　75 歳女性
	(英語)	24	CASE22　30-year-old woman
	(英語)	25	CASE23　75-year-old woman

目次 Index

英日マークは英語・日本語，英マークは英語が CD に録音されています．

PART 1　Communication 編 ... 1

受付・検査室・診療科での会話例 ... 4
共通問診 ... 7

内　科 ... 11

パターン 1　症状はありますか ... 12
パターン 2　症状や原因を尋ねる ... 16
　英日 Case 1-1　急性胃炎（34 歳女性） ... 18
パターン 3　診察時の会話 ... 20
　英日 Case 1-2　急性胃炎（34 歳女性） ... 21
パターン 4　痛みについて詳しく尋ねる ... 23
パターン 5　痛みがいつ（when），どこ（where），どのくらい（how）起こるかを尋ねる ... 25
　英日 Case 2-1　狭心症（54 歳男性） ... 27
　Case 2-2　狭心症（54 歳男性）検査後 ... 30
パターン 6　～するために，治療・検査・手術が必要でしょう ... 32
パターン 7　検査の結果，（診断など）であることがわかりました ... 32
パターン 8　～のリスクについて説明する ... 33
パターン 9　安全であることを伝える ... 34
　英日 Case 3　糖尿病（45 歳男性） ... 35
パターン 10　1. 病気／症状は～が原因でしょう
　　　　　　　　2. ～が，病気／症状の原因でしょう ... 37
　英 Case 4-1　頚部リンパ節腫脹（28 歳女性） ... 38
　英 Case 4-2　頚部リンパ節腫脹（28 歳女性）：歯科受診 ... 40
パターン 11　指示 1　～を取ってください，～を避けてください，薬などを出しましょう ... 44
パターン 12　指示 2　～するとよいでしょう．ぜひ～しましょう ... 46
パターン 13　紹介状を書く ... 46
　英日 Case 5　高血圧症（66 歳女性） ... 47

目 次

小児科 — 49

パターン1	子供の症状を家族に尋ねる	
	症状があったようですか	50
パターン2	診断・検査・指示などによく用いる主文導入部のフレーズ(1)	52
パターン3	主文導入部のフレーズ(2)	53
パターン4	症状が認められますか	53
パターン5	随伴症状を別の言い方で尋ねる	53
英日 Case 6-1	腸重積症(生後11ヵ月男児)	55
英日 Case 6-2	腸重積症(生後11ヵ月男児)	56
パターン6	診察時の会話	58
英日 Case 7-1	インフルエンザ(7歳女児)	59
パターン7	指示	61
英 Case 7-2	インフルエンザ(7歳女児)	64
パターン8	授乳についての問診	66
英 Case 8-1	尿路感染症(生後5ヵ月男児)	67
英 Case 8-2	尿路感染症(生後5ヵ月男児)	68
Case 8-3	尿路感染症(生後5ヵ月男児)	69
パターン9	健診時の問診	71
英日 Case 9-1	乳幼児健診(生後10ヵ月男児)	72
パターン10	健診時の指示	73
Case 9-2	乳幼児健診(生後10ヵ月男児)	73
パターン11	予防接種時の会話	75
英日 Case 10-1	流行性耳下腺炎(5歳男児)	76
Case 10-2	流行性耳下腺炎(5歳男児)	77
Case 10-3	流行性耳下腺炎(5歳男児)	78

産婦人科 — 81

パターン1	症状について尋ねる	82
パターン2	月経／出血についての問診	83
英 Case 11-1	不正出血(26歳女性)	85
英 Case 11-2	不正出血(26歳女性)	87
パターン3	妊娠歴／避妊についての問診	89
英日 Case 12-1	卵巣嚢腫(34歳女性)	90
英日 Case 12-2	卵巣嚢腫(34歳女性)	91
パターン4	診察時の会話	93

ix

英	Case 12-3	卵巣嚢腫(34歳女性)	94
パターン5		帯下についての問診	96
英日	Case 13	腟炎(41歳女性)	97

整形外科 — 99

パターン1		～する時, ～(部位)が～の状態ですか	100
パターン2		～すると(～する時), 悪化しますか	102
パターン3		～できますか	103
英日	Case 14	上腕骨骨折(20歳男性)	105
英日	Case 15-1	腰椎椎間板ヘルニア(32歳男性)	107
英	Case 15-2	腰椎椎間板ヘルニア(32歳男性)	108
パターン4		診察時の会話	109
英日	Case 16-1	骨粗鬆症(75歳女性)	110
英	Case 16-2	骨粗鬆症(75歳女性)	112
パターン5		指示	114
英日	Case 17	手根管症候群(24歳女性)	115

皮膚科 — 117

パターン1		問診	118
英日	Case 18-1	薬剤アレルギー(薬疹)(50歳男性)	120
英日	Case 18-2	薬剤アレルギー(薬疹)(50歳男性)	121
英日	Case 19-1	アトピー性皮膚炎(22歳女性)	123
英	Case 19-2	アトピー性皮膚炎(22歳女性)	124

眼　科 — 127

パターン1		問診1　どちらが～ですか	128
パターン2		問診2	129
	Case 20	麦粒腫(30歳男性)	131
	Case 21	角膜異物(40歳男性)	132
英日	Case 22	網膜剥離(30歳女性)	134
英日	Case 23	急性緑内障発作(75歳女性)	135

PART 2　Basic Medical Writing 編　　137

- A. 基本的な Writing Patterns を紹介します …………………………………………………… 138
- B. Case Report を書いてみましょう …………………………………………………………… 143

[Case 1]	胃潰瘍	143	[Case 15]	手根管症候群	149
[Case 2-1]	ウイルス性急性肝炎	143	[Case 16]	小児弾撥指	149
[Case 2-2]	ウイルス性急性肝炎	143	[Case 17]	足底腱膜炎	149
[Case 3]	胃癌	144	[Case 18]	有痛性外脛骨	150
[Case 4]	急性胃炎	144	[Case 19-1]	左胸背部帯状疱疹	150
[Case 5-1]	川崎病	144	[Case 19-2]	左胸背部帯状疱疹	150
[Case 5-2]	川崎病	145	[Case 20-1]	アレルギー性紫斑病	150
[Case 6-1]	気管支喘息	145	[Case 20-2]	アレルギー性紫斑病	151
[Case 6-2]	気管支喘息	145	[Case 21-1]	悪性黒色腫：皮膚生検	151
[Case 7]	左外鼠径ヘルニア（嵌頓）	146	[Case 21-2]	悪性黒色腫：皮膚生検	152
[Case 8]	突発性発疹	146	[Case 22-1]	皮脂欠乏性湿疹	152
[Case 9]	カンジダ腟炎	146	[Case 22-2]	皮脂欠乏性湿疹	152
[Case 10]	子宮内膜症	147	[Case 23]	近視	153
[Case 11]	子宮外妊娠	147	[Case 24]	弱視	153
[Case 12]	バルトリン腺膿瘍	147	[Case 25]	急性結膜浮腫	153
[Case 13]	クラミジア子宮頸管炎	148	[Case 26]	眼底出血	153
[Case 14]	更年期障害	148	[Case 27]	ぶどう膜炎（虹彩毛様体脈絡膜炎）	154

● 解答編（別冊）

CD レコーディングスタッフ　（声の出演）

Julia Summerhill
Robert Conroy
大橋　正幸（学校法人コンピュータ総合学園神戸電子専門学校／声優タレント学科教員）
松本雄太朗（学校法人コンピュータ総合学園神戸電子専門学校／声優タレント学科）
川上あゆみ（学校法人コンピュータ総合学園神戸電子専門学校／声優タレント学科）

Recording & Engineering

Studio Neko　小林弘明

PART 1
Communication 編

- 内　科　11
- 小児科　49
- 産婦人科　81
- 整形外科　99
- 皮膚科　117
- 眼　科　127

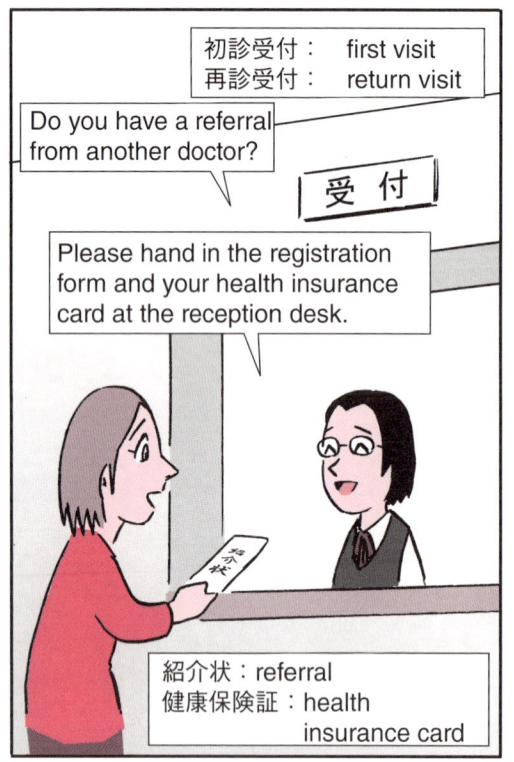
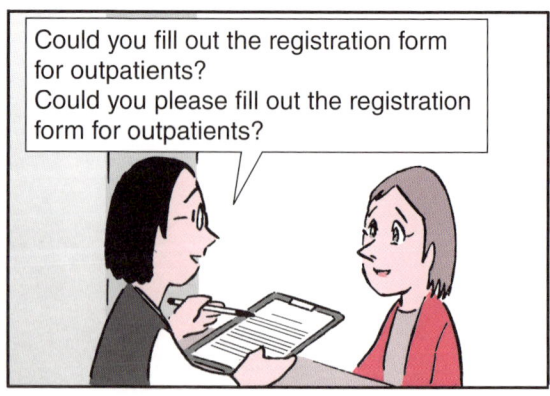
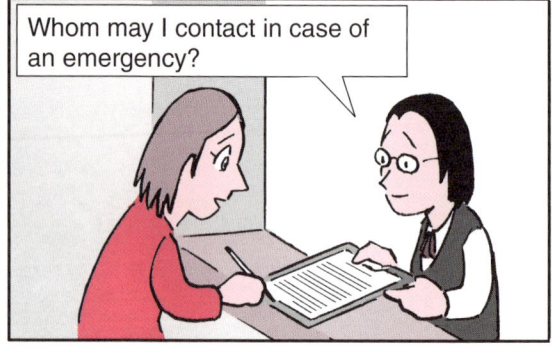
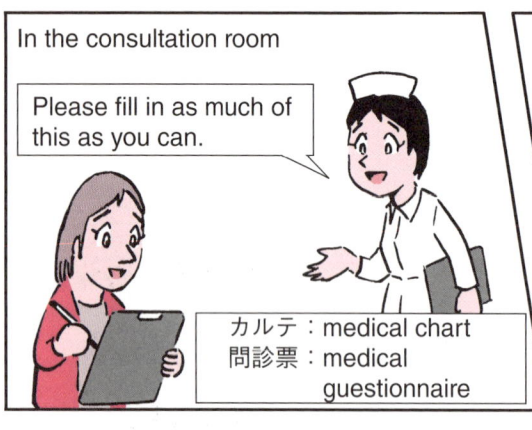
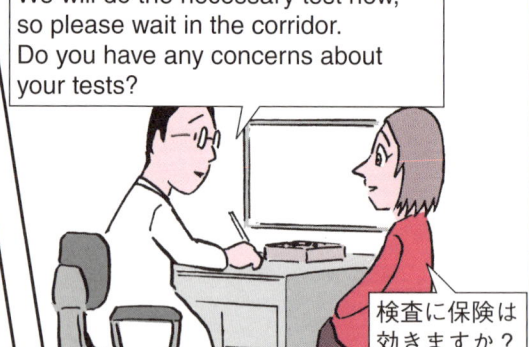
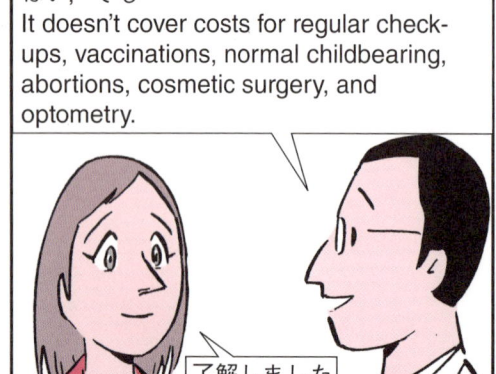
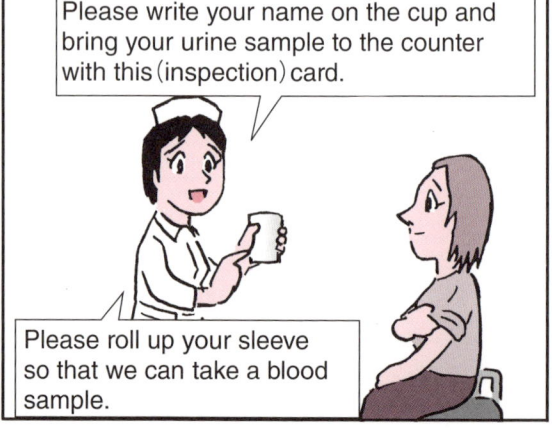

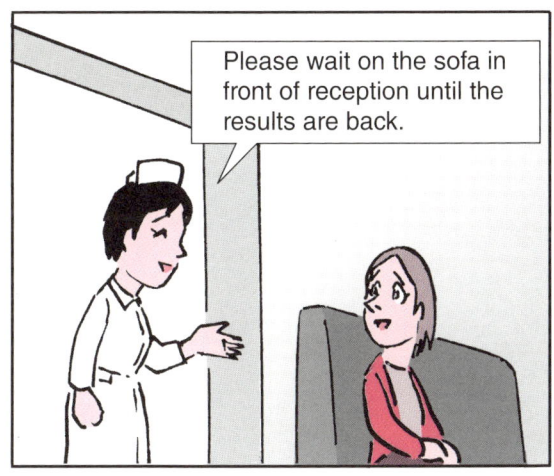
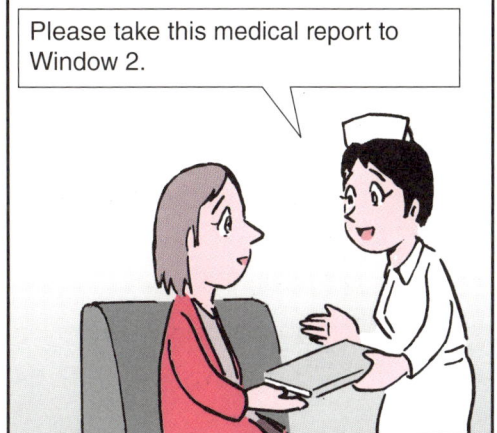
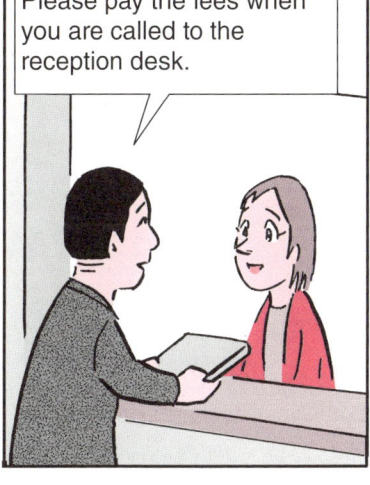
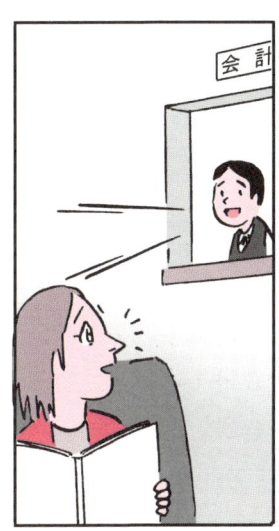
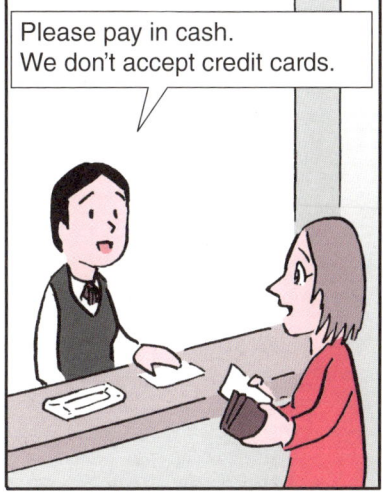
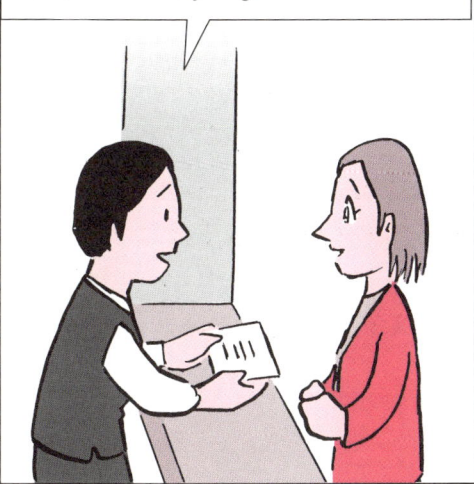
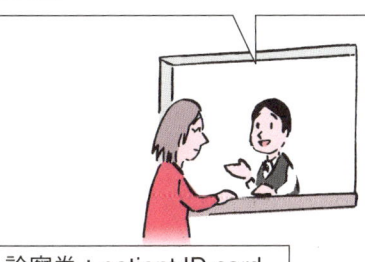

診察券：patient ID card

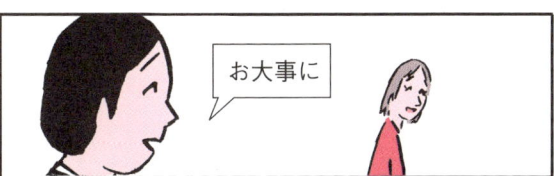

受付・検査室・診療科での会話例

受付

健康保険証 health insurance card
診察券 patient ID card
カルテ medical chart
問診票 medical questionnaire
再診受付 return visit

Could you fill out the registration form for outpatients?（外来患者用の診察問診票に記入していただけませんか．）

Please hand in the registration form and your health insurance card at the reception desk.（申込書と健康保険証を受付に提出してください．）

Whom may I contact in case of an emergency?（緊急の場合はどなたに連絡を取ればいいですか．）

Do you have a referral from another doctor?（医師の紹介状をお持ちですか．）

Please be sure to bring your health insurance card the first time you come in a month.（月の最初の診察時には健康保険証を必ずお持ちください．）

It doesn't cover the cost of regular check-ups, vaccinations, normal childbearing, abortions, cosmetic surgery, or optometry.（健康診断，予防接種，普通分娩，妊娠中絶，美容整形や視力測定などは，健康保険の対象になりません．）

Please do not forget to bring your patient ID card.（診察券を忘れずにお持ちください．）

Please fill in as much of this as you can.（問診票にわかる範囲で記入してください．）

Please pay the fee when you are called to the reception desk.（お名前が呼ばれましたら受付で料金をお支払いください．）

Please pay the fee at the reception desk.（受付で料金をお支払いください．）

Please pay in cash.（現金でお支払いください．）

We don't accept credit cards.（クレジットカードではお支払いいただけません．）

Please go to the XX Pharmacy to have your prescription filled.（XX薬局に行って処方箋の薬を受け取ってください．）

(Note: 名前を入れない場合，a pharmacy になります．小文字を使います．)

検査室

We will do the necessary tests now, so please wait in the corridor.（今から必要な検査を行いますので，廊下でお待ちください．）

Do you have any concerns about your tests?（検査について何か心配なことはありますか．）

Please wait on the sofa in reception until the results are ready.（結果が分かるまで，受付のソファでお待ちください．）

Please write your name on the cup and bring your urine sample to the counter with this (inspection) card.〔Urine test〕（コップに名前を書いて，尿サンプルを検査票といっしょにカウンターにお出し下さい．）

Please roll up your sleeve so that we can take a blood sample.〔Blood test〕（血液サンプルを取りますのでそでを上げて下さい．）

Please submit this medical report to Window 2.（カルテを2番の窓口にお出しください．）

診療科

　　一般内科 General Internal Medicine
　　呼吸器内科 Respiratory Medicine
　　循環器内科 Cardiology
　　消化器内科 Gastroenterology
　　内分泌代謝科 Endocrinology and Metabolism
　　血液内科 Hematology
　　心療内科 Psychosomatic Medicine
　　一般外科 General Surgery
　　呼吸器外科 Thoracic Surgery
　　心臓外科 Cardiovascular Surgery
　　乳腺外科 Breast Surgery
　　内分泌外科 Endocrine Surgery
　　整形外科 Orthopedic Surgery
　　形成外科 Plastic Surgery
　　脳神経外科 Neurosurgery
　　小児外科 Pediatric Surgery
　　小児科 Pediatrics
　　産科婦人科 Obstetrics and Gynecology
　　泌尿器科 Urology
　　皮膚科 Dermatology

眼科 Ophthalmology
耳鼻咽喉科 Otorhinolaryngology, ENT
精神科 Psychiatry
放射線科 Radiology
歯科 Dentistry
口腔外科 Oral Surgery
救急救命室：Emergency Department（ED）, Accident & Emergency（A&E）, Emergency Room（ER）, Emergency Ward（EW）

共通問診

> ～はありますか．Is there～　Do you have ～
> ～はありましたか．Were there ～
> ～したことはありますか．Have you ever had ～
> どのくらいの頻度で～ですか．How often do you ～
> ～は飲んでいますか．Are you taking ～

主訴 Chief Complaints(CC)

Do you have any *weakness*, *dizziness*, or *fainting*? *Fatigue* or *weight loss*?

随伴症状

Do you have any accompanying symptoms, such as ~?

Are there any associated symptoms?

内服薬 Medications(MEDS)

Are you taking any prescription or nonprescription medicines?（何か処方薬か市販薬をのんでいますか．）

What is the dose and frequency?

Have you recently increased the dose of any medicine?

How well have they worked?（どんな風に効果がありましたか．）

現病歴 History of Present Illness(HPI)

Are there any medical conditions you have now or used to have?（現在，またはこれまでに何か病気をしましたか．）

What treatments have you tried?

Is the problem getting better, worse, or staying the same?

既往歴 Past Medical History(PMH)

Is there/Do you have a(any) history of *constipation*?

Have you ever had this happen before?

Have you ever been diagnosed with *hypertension*?

Have you ever had any major illness or any bad injuries?（何か大きな病気かけがをしたことはありますか．）

Were there any complications?（合併症はありましたか．）

手術歴 Past Surgical History (PSH)

Have you ever had any operations?（これまでに何か手術をしたことがありますか．）

Have you been operated on, even as a child?

Have you ever been hospitalized for any operations?

家族歴 Family History (FH)

Do you have a family history of *cancer*?

Does anyone in your family have ▢ a ▢ ?（ご家族で〜の人はいますか．）

▶ a に以下の言葉を入れてみましょう．

high blood pressure 高血圧　　　　high blood sugar 高血糖
any serious illness 何か大きな病気
what you have now 今あなたがかかっている病気
problems with mental health, such as depression うつのような精神的な病気

Does anyone in your family have problems with *mental health, such as depression*? （注：かぜ等の一過性の疾患の場合は，既往歴・家族歴などはあまり重要でない場合が多いが，心疾患・呼吸器疾患などの場合にはこれらの聴取も重要）

アレルギー Allergies/Reactions (ALL/RXNs)

Do you have any allergies?

Do you have any allergies to ▢ b ▢ ?（〜にアレルギーはありますか．）

▶ b に以下の言葉を入れてみましょう．

prescription medication 処方薬　　　food 食べ物
animals 動物　　　　　　　　　　　plants 植物

Are you allergic to *any medications like penicillin* (or have you had adverse reactions to drugs, anesthesia or food in the past)? If so, why were you taking it and what was your reaction?

渡航歴 Travel / 接触歴

Have you recently traveled outside the country?

Have you recently been exposed to someone with a similar illness?

Have you had contact with anyone who has had *tuberculosis*?

生活歴（喫煙・アルコール摂取）Social History (SH) (Smoking/Alcohol Intake)

Do you drink alcohol? If so, how much?

Do you smoke (cigarettes)? If so, how many? What kind?

Do you smoke very little, or is it many years since you last smoked?

食事(Diet)

Has there been any recent change in your weight?（最近体重が変わりましたか．）
Are you on any special diet?（何か特別なダイエットはしていますか．）

睡眠・ストレス(Sleep・stress)

Do you tend to get stressed easily?（ストレスを受けやすいですか．）
Do you think you're getting enough sleep?（十分な睡眠がとれていると思いますか．）
Has there been any change in how much you sleep?（睡眠時間に何か変化はありますか．）
Have you had any stressful events recently?（最近何かストレスになるような事がありますか．）
Are you having any stress from work?（仕事で何かストレスがありますか．）
Is there any stress at home?（ご家庭で何かストレスはありますか．）

排尿(Urination)

Do you have any problem with urination?（排尿に何か問題はありますか．）
How often do you urinate?（何回ぐらいおしっこをしますか．）
How many times do you get up at night to urinate?（おしっこで何回ぐらい夜起きますか．）
Do you have any burning sensation with urination?（おしっこをすると，焼けるような感覚がありますか．）
Does your water burn when you have to pass it?
Is the burning present throughout the stream?
Any blood?（血は混ざっていますか．）

健康保険(Health insurance)

Do you have health insurance for your husband?
What type of insurance is your new baby covered by?

病気による影響について尋ねる

Does your problem interfere with your job or household responsibilities?
Does your problem make it difficult for you to do strenuous housework?
Does your problem make it difficult for you to walk by yourself?
Does your problem make it difficult for you to concentrate?
Because of your problem, are you depressed?
How has that affected you?

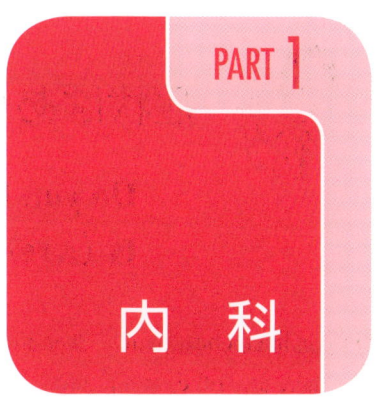

PART 1

内 科

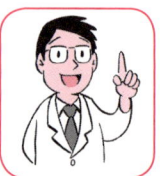

パターン1
症状はありますか

1 **Do you have** 症 状 ?
2 **Is (Are) there** 症 状 ?

Do you have chest pain?　胸痛がありますか.
Are there any other symptoms?　その他に症状はありますか.

Do you have <u>a rash</u> ＋ <u>with fever</u> ＋ <u>after eating shrimp</u>?
　　　　　　症状　　　　随伴症状　　　　　　　　いつ
エビを食べた後, 熱を伴って発疹がでましたか。

[英会話文の基本的な骨格]

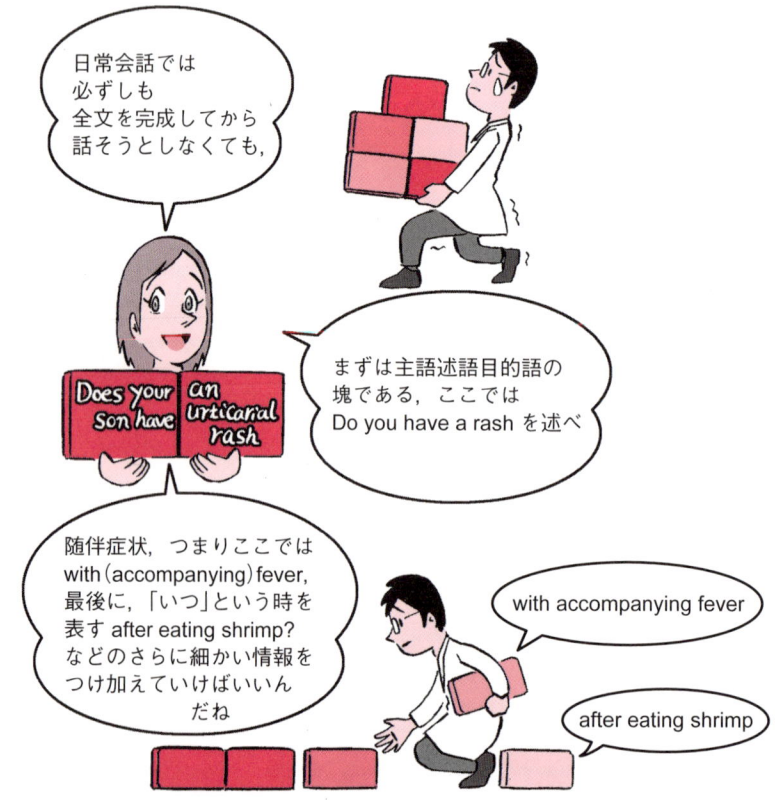

Easy Talk !　英文の特徴として,
1　一番伝えたい重要な内容[SVO 誰がどうした何を]の塊を最初にのべ,
2　そのあとに「随伴症状」「いつ」などの less important な情報を順番に足していきます。

内　科

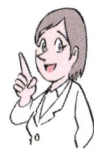

使えるパターンを増やそう！

〜すると（時），症状がありますか

Do you have 　症　状　 + when 〜？

例　Do you have an abdominal pain ＋ when your stomach is empty?
　　お腹がすくと（すいている時），お腹が痛みますか．

あてはめましょう！

次の枠内に(a)〜(c)の用語をあてはめて，症状を尋ねてください．

(a)　Do you have ☐ ?
(b)　Are (Is) there ☐ ?
(c)　Does ☐ have high sugar levels or heart disease?

(a)　nausea or vomiting 吐き気または嘔吐，loss of appetite 食欲不振
(b)　chest pain 胸痛，palpitations 動悸，dyspnea 呼吸困難，pedal edema 足の浮腫，syncope 失神，nocturia or dysuria 夜間頻尿または排尿障害，heavy chest pressure　胸が圧迫されるような感じ
(c)　anyone in your family ご家族で誰か

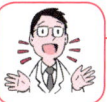

練　習　このパターンでこれだけ話せる！　　　　　（解答は別冊）

1. 咳をすると，胸が痛みますか．
2. 階段を上る時，足の痛みはありますか．
3. 横になると，息苦しくなりますか．
4. 激しい運動をすると，息切れしますか．
5. 息をする時，ゼーゼーいいますか．
6. 運動すると，ふらつきますか．
7. しばらく食べていないと，ふらつきますか．
8. 眩暈がする時，ふらつきますか．

13

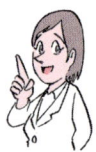

使えるパターンを増やそう！

病名・家族歴・既往歴を尋ねる

Do you have ＋ ① disease 病　名 ?
② a history of 既往歴 ?
③ a family history of 家族歴 ?

症状の代わりに，病名・家族歴・既往歴などに置き換えることができます．

例 1　Do you have diabetes?　糖尿病はありますか．
例 2　Do you have a history of food allergies?　食べ物のアレルギーの既往歴はありますか．
例 3　Do you have a family history of heart disease?　ご家族で心臓病の人はいますか．

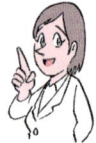

使えるパターンを増やそう！

既往歴を別の言い方で尋ねる
これまでに〜したことはありますか

Have you ever had 病 名・症 状・手 術 ?
Have you ever been told that you have 病 名 ?

例 1　Have you ever experienced（had）a heart attack?
　　　これまでに心臓発作を起こしたことはありますか．
例 2　Have you ever been told you have diabetes?
　　　これまでに糖尿病と言われたことはありますか．

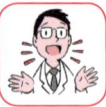

練 習　このパターンでこれだけ話せる　　　　　　　（解答は別冊）

9. これまでにリウマチ熱があると言われたことはありますか．
10. これまでに甲状腺疾患がありますか
11. これまでに立ち上がった時，意識を失ったり，バランスを崩したことがありますか．
12. これまで咳のために目が覚めたことはありますか．
13. これまでに胸の圧迫感や不整脈はありましたか．
14. これまでに心臓カテーテル検査や心臓手術を受けたことはありますか．
15. これまで喘鳴を自覚したことがありますか．
16. これまで健康に何か変化がありましたか．

【ヒント】　リウマチ熱 rheumatic fever，甲状腺疾患 thyroid problems，心臓カテーテル cardiac catheterization

内　科

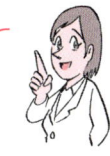

使えるパターンを増やそう！

Do you have 症　状 ?

例文の"have"を他の動詞に置き換えることができます．
① **have**：慢性的な症状がある
② **feel**：症状を感じる
③ **experience**：症状を経験したことがある
④ **get**：症状が始まる，〜になる
⑤ **notice**：症状に気づく

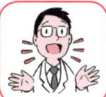

練　習　このパターンでこれだけ話せる！　　（解答は別冊）

17. 最後にこの痛みが起きたのはいつごろですか．
18. この痛みをいつごろ感じましたか．
19. この痛みはいつごろ始まりましたか．
20. 尿に血が混ざっているのに初めて気がついたのはいつごろですか．
21. ぐるぐる回る感じですか．
22. どちらかに傾く感じはありますか．

これらの動詞のイメージを説明します．実際には慣用的に用いられているので，会話をする上では，フレーズとして言い慣れることが有効でしょう．

① **have**：慢性的な症状がある場合，現在もある場合に用います．また，眩暈，パニックなどが起きて，現在治まっている場合も用います．
　　have a pain　痛みが（ずっと，いまも）ある．
　　have dizzy spells　眩暈がする．
　　have panic attacks　パニック発作がある．

② **feel**：患者さんが感じた経験を述べる時に用います．
　　feel pain, dizzy, nausea, headache, faint　痛み・めまい・吐き気・頭痛がある・気を失う．

③ **experience**：これも同様に用いることができますが，attacks（発作）など患者さんが瞬間に経験した場合に用います．長期的な a rash（発疹）には，普通用いません．
　　experience pain, dizzy, nausea, headache, attacks　痛み・めまい・吐き気・頭痛・発作が起きることがある．

④ **get**：過去に起きていて，症状が始まった時に用います．
　　get rashes, dizzy　発疹が出始める，めまいが始まる．

⑤ **notice**：気づく
　　notice blood, clots, numbness　血・血塊・しびれに気がつく．

15

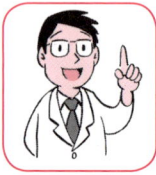

パターン 2
症状や原因を尋ねる

◉様子

1. What kind of 症状 is it?　症状は，どのような感じですか
   What does 症状 feel like?/Would you please describe 症状 ?
   なども使います．

◉原因

2. What do you think causes 症状・病気 ?
   何か症状を引き起こすような原因に心当たりがありますか．

3. What makes 症状・病気 worse or better? For example, 〜
   何かのきっかけで，症状がひどくなったり，よくなったりしますか．たとえば〜

例1　What kind of pain is it? Gnawing or stabbing?
　　　痛みは，どのような感じですか．しくしくするような痛みとかきりきりするとか．

例2　What makes your pain worse? For example, eating fatty food or drinking alcohol?
　　　何かのきっかけで，痛みがひどくなりますか，たとえば，脂っこい食事をするとかお酒を飲むとか．

例3　What makes your pain better? For example, eating food or taking drugs?
　　　何かすると，痛みが和らぎますか，たとえば，食べ物を食べるとか，薬を飲むとか．

内 科

Words & expressions　痛みの様子・程度を表す表現例

sharp 鋭い，dull 鈍い，mild 軽い，severe 激しい
gnawing しくしくする（例：gnawing abdominal pain）
gripping きりきり刺すような（例：gripping pain in my chest/stomach）
throbbing ずきずきするような（例：throbbing headache 拍動痛）
stabbing 刺すような（例：stabbing pain 刺痛）
crushing ずきずきするような（例：crushing chest pain）
cramping 痙性（例：menstrual cramping 生理痛）
colicky 疝痛の（例：colicky abdominal pain 疝痛性腹痛）
persistent/constant 持続性の，intermittent 間欠的な，periodic 周期性の

Words & expressions　症状を悪化させるきっかけとなる表現例

eating fatty food 脂肪分の多い食べ物を取る
drinking 飲酒，smoking 喫煙，taking NSAIDs 非ステロイド系消炎鎮痛剤を飲む
being under stress ストレスがある，climbing stairs 階段を上る
walking fast 速く歩く，exposure to pollen 花粉にさらされる
exposure to sunlight 日光にあたる，exposure to cold air 冷たい空気にさらす
changes in temperature 気温の変化，moving about 動き回る

Words & expressions　症状を改善するきっかけとなる例

having a/some rest 休息を取る，taking drugs 薬を飲む，keeping still 動かない
moving around 動き回る，acupuncture and moxibustion 鍼や灸
massage マッサージ

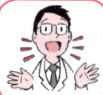

練習　このパターンで，これだけ話せる！　　　　（解答は別冊）

23. どのようにしたら腫れがひきますか．
24. お腹が痛くなるような原因に何か心当たりはありませんか．たとえば，生肉，卵や魚などの生ものを食べたとか．海外旅行をしたとか．
25. 胸の痛みはどんな痛みですか．たとえば，圧迫されるようなとか，重い感じとか．
26. 朝晩に痛みはひどくなりますか．
27. 休息時，運動をしている時，ストレスがある時，食後，腕を動かした後に痛みがおこりますか．
28. 眩暈を起こす可能性のあるものに何か心当たりはありませんか．

Case 1-1　急性胃炎(34歳女性)

- Dr. Hello. What seems to be the problem today?
- Pt. I have a stomach ache.
- Dr. Can you point out exactly where it hurts?
- Pt. Around here 〔*stroking the epigastric area*〕
- Dr. There? Do you feel pain now?
- Pt. Yes, a little bit.
- Dr. What kind of pain is it? For example, is it burning, stabbing, gnawing, cramping, sharp, or dull?
- Pt. Well, I have a bit of a heavy pain. When it gets worse, it is more of a stabbing pain.
- Dr. Does it come and go?
- Pt. Yes.
- Dr. When did it start?
- Pt. I have had a somewhat uncomfortable feeling in my stomach for about a week. It has been getting worse since yesterday.
- Dr. When do you feel pain? For example, when your stomach is empty or after a meal?
- Pt. Mostly it hurts when my stomach is empty. It is most intense first thing in the morning.
- Dr. Does the pain get worse when you eat greasy food?
- Pt. Umm… No, I don't think so.
- Dr. Have you ever had any serious illnesses or diseases? Are you taking any medicine?
- Pt. No.

- Dr. こんにちは，今日はどうされましたか．
- Pt. おなかが痛みます．
- Dr. 一番痛いところはどのあたりですか．
- Pt. このあたりです．〔上腹部をなでながら〕
- Dr. そこですか．今も痛みますか．
- Pt. はい．少し．
- Dr. どのような痛みですか．例えば，焼きつくようなとか，きりきりとか，しくしくとか，けいれん性，鋭いとか鈍いとか．
- Pt. そうですね．少し重い感じで，ひどい時は，きりきりと痛みます．
- Dr. それは，痛くなったり，良くなったりしますか．
- Pt. そうです．

Dr.	いつから痛み始めましたか．	Dr.	脂っぽいものを食べると，痛みはひどくなりますか．
Pt.	一週間前ぐらいから，おなかに幾分不快感がありました．昨日から，ひどくなっています．	Pt.	えっと，そうでもないです．
Dr.	いつ痛みますか．例えば，空腹時とか食後とか．	Dr.	今までに，何か大きな病気をしたことがありますか．また，今何か薬を飲んでいますか．
Pt.	たいていは，空腹時です．朝が一番痛みます．	Pt.	いいえ．

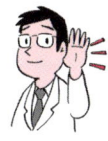

[Listening comprehension]　　　　　　　（解答は別冊）

29. What is the patient's chief complaint?
30. What kind of pain does he have when it gets worse? Choose the correct one.

  A. heavy B. burning C. stabbing
  D. throbbing E. cramping

📌 **メディカルコーナー：熱やその他の症状を尋ねる時**

①熱について，体温は測定の結果でわかるので，患者さんには以下のように問診します．
「熱っぽいですか」 "Do you feel feverish?" 「家で，熱を測りましたか」 "Have you taken your temperature at home?"

②症状を尋ねる時は，「呼吸器症状」 "respiratory symptoms" のような専門用語は用いないようにします．「咳がありますか．痰は出ますか」 "Do you have a cough? Do you bring up any sputum?" など具体的に尋ねます．

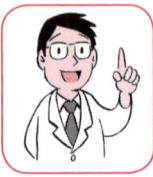

パターン3 診察時の会話

1 Please remove your clothes from the waist up (down)...
上(下)半身の服を脱いでください．

Please pull down your underwear and show me your abdomen.
下着を下げて，おなかを見せてください．

Let me take a look at your throat. 喉をみましょう．

Please expose your abdomen. お腹を出してください．

2 Now breathe deeply while I listen to your chest.... breathe in.... out.... in.... out.... OK.
それでは，胸の音を聞きますから，息を深く吸ってください．吸って，吐いて，吸って，吐いて，いいですよ．

Please take a deep breath in. Hold it, and relax.
深く息を吸って，止めて，はい，いいですよ．

3 I'd like to see your back, so please turn around.
背中をみますから，後ろを向いてください．

4 Please lie down on your back on the examination table with your legs bent at the knees/with your knees bent.
診察台に仰向けに寝て，膝を立ててください．

Lie face up with your legs straight. Lie on your left side.
仰向けに寝て，足を伸ばしてください．体の左側を下にして横になってください．

5 You may get dressed now. 服を着ていいですよ．

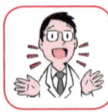

練 習 このパターンでこれだけ話せる！　　　（解答は別冊）

31. ベッドに仰向けに寝て膝を立ててください．
32. うつぶせに寝てください．
33. ベルトを緩めて，パンツを下げてください．
34. こちら側を頭にして，仰向けに休んでいただけますか．
35. 左側を下にして横になってください．

Case 1-2　急性胃炎（34歳女性）

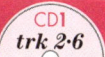

- **Dr.** I see. Now I am going to examine your stomach. Please lie flat on your back with your legs bent at the knees. Do you feel pain here?（Does it hurt?）〔*Palpating the abdomen*〕
- **Pt.** No.
- **Dr.** How about here?
- **Pt.** Ouch! When you push, it hurts. But it hurts more on the right side of that spot.
- **Dr.** Around here?
- **Pt.** Yes, that's the most painful spot.
- **Dr.** 〔*While palpating*〕Does it hurt when I tap it like this?... OK, please get up and put on your clothes.
  〔*The patient gets dressed*〕
- **Dr.** Well, the most likely diagnosis would be acute gastritis. Other likely possibilities include gastric ulcer and pancreatitis.
  Gastric cancer cannot be ruled out, although it is a rare diagnosis. For the time being, I will give you medications for gastritis and gastric ulcers. Please do not take stimulants such as coffee. And please chew your food well. This helps not just to break the food down well, but also mixes the food with saliva. It reduces the burden on the digestive system.
  You also need to have an endoscopy to rule out gastric cancer.
- **Pt.** Endoscopy? I'd rather not have that procedure.
- **Dr.** If it's early-stage stomach cancer, it nearly always can be cured. So, is that OK with you?
- **Pt.** Alright.
- **Dr.** Please do not eat or drink, except for tea or water, after supper on the day before the examination.

- **Dr.** わかりました．さあ，おなかを診ましょう．ベッドに横になって，膝を立ててください．〔*お腹を触診をしながら*〕ここは痛いですか．
- **Pt.** いいえ．
- **Dr.** ここはどうですか．
- **Pt.** あ，痛い！抑えられた時，痛みます．でも，その右の方がもっと痛みます．
- **Dr.** このあたりですか．

Pt. はい，そこが最も痛いところです．
Dr. 〔触診中に〕このようにたたくと痛みますか．
いいですよ．起きて洋服を着てください．
〔患者が服を着る〕
Dr. そうですね，急性胃炎の可能性がもっとも高いですが，胃潰瘍や，膵炎の可能性もあります．
稀ですが，胃癌の可能性も否定できません．とりあえず，胃炎や胃潰瘍に効く薬を出しましょう．コーヒーや刺激物はとらないでください．食べ物はよく噛んでください．食べ物をよく砕くだけでなく，唾液と食べ物をよく混ぜるのにも役立ちます．その結果，消化器系への負担を減らします．癌でないことを確認するために，胃カメラもする必要があります．
Pt. 胃カメラですか．やりたくないです．
Dr. 早期がんであればほとんど助かります．ですから，胃カメラをしましょう．
Pt. わかりました．
Dr. 検査前日の夕食後は，水とお茶以外は，飲んだり食べたりしないでください．

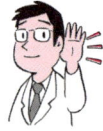

[Listening comprehension]

（解答は別冊）

36. What is the most likely diagnosis? Choose the correct one.
 A. chronic gastritis B. acute gastritis
 C. pancreatitis D. gastric cancer

📌 **文法コーナー　lay と lie の用法**

・lay は他動詞で目的語をとりますが，lie は自動詞で目的語をとりません．Lay（〜を置く）の現在形と lie（横たわる）の過去形が同じ lay なので紛らわしいところです．

現在形	過去形	過去分詞	
lie	lay	lain	横になる　横たわる．
lay	laid	laid	〜を置く・〜をもたれかける．

Please lie down on the bed. ベッドに横になってください．
Yesterday I lay down all day. 昨日は一日中，横になっていました．
I have lain down at home since then それ以後，家でゴロゴロしています．
Every day, I lay the key on the table. いつも鍵をテーブルに置きます．
Yesterday, he laid the key on the table. 昨日，彼は鍵をテーブルの上に置いておきました．
He has laid the key on the table after he brought it back. 彼は，鍵を持ち帰ったあと，テーブルの上に置いておきました．

内　科

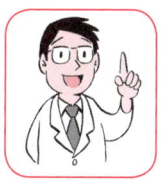

パターン4
痛みについて詳しく尋ねる
痛みは〜ですか

Does the pain 〜?

1 Does the pain come on slowly or suddenly?
痛みは徐々に起こりますか，それとも急に起こりますか．

Did the pain come on slowly or suddenly?
痛みは徐々に起こりましたか，それとも突然起こりましたか（現在痛みが消えている場合）

2 Does the pain go away/subside?　今は，もう痛みは消えましたか．

Does it still hurt now?　まだ痛みますか．

3 Does the pain come and go?　痛みが起こったり，消えたりしますか．

Is the pain constant or intermittent?
痛みはずっと継続しますか，それとも出たり出なかったりしますか．

4 Does the pain radiate to your arms or face?
痛みは，腕や顔まで走りますか．
radiate to の代わりに，spread to/move to なども使います．

5 Does it hurt ＋ when I push here or when I relieve the pressure?
ここを押さえると痛みますか．それとも，手を離した時痛みますか．
Dose it hurt の代わりに，Is it painful ともいえます．

Does the pain occur ＋ before, during or after meals?
痛みは，食事前，食事中，または，食後に起こりますか．

［ポイント1］　"the pain" をその他の症状に置き換えることもできます．

例　Does the rash usually spread to your arms or face?　発赤はいつも腕や顔まで広がりますか．

Easy talk!
"Does the pain" "Does it hurt" などは，"one word" のように話しましょう．

23

Easy talk!　the pain を it に置き換えると幅広く症状を尋ねることができます．
例　How long have you had it?　どれくらいの間，その症状は続いていますか．
短文は文全体を長い一語のつもりで言いましょう．

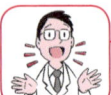

練習　このパターンでこれだけ話せる！　　（解答は別冊）

37. 痛みは腰に広がりますか．
38. 発赤は他の場所に広がりますか．
39. ここを押さえて手を離したら痛みますか．
40. 痛みは急に始まりますか，それとも徐々に痛くなりますか．
41. めまいはずっとありますか，それとも突然起こりますか．

用語・用法の研究　部位別の痛み

腰の痛みは，pain in your lower back より lower back pain を用います．同様に，腕や足の痛み（arms and leg pain）を尋ねる場合，"Do you have pain in your arms and legs?" の代わりに，"Do you have any leg pain?" または "Do you have any arm pain?" などとも言えます．

---

words & expressions

頭痛	headache	のどの痛み	sore throat
胸痛	chest pain	歯痛	toothache
腹痛	abdominal pain	筋肉痛	sore muscles
胃痛	stomach ache	関節痛	joint pain

内　科

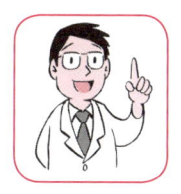

パターン5
痛みがいつ(when)，どこ(where)，どのくらい(how)起こるかを尋ねる

When does the pain 〜?
Where is the pain（located）?
How does the pain 〜?

● [いつ]

1　When **did the pain** start?　いつ痛みだしましたか．

　　When were you last completely well?　いつ痛みが完全になくなりましたか．

2　When **does the pain** occur?　いつ痛みますか．

　　For example, at rest?　静かにしている時ですか．
　　　　　　　　　–while exercising?　運動している時ですか．
　　　　　　　　　–after exertion?　運動後ですか．
　　　　　　　　　–when climbing stairs?　階段を登る時ですか．
　　　　　　　　　–when lying flat/down or sitting up?
　　　　　　　　　　　　　横になった時に苦しいですか．それとも，座った時ですか．

3　When **does the pain** get better?　いつ痛みがよくなりますか．

　　When **does the pain** get worse?　いつ痛みがひどくなりますか．

● [どこ]

4　Where **does it hurt?**　どこが痛みますか．

　　Where is the pain（located）?

● [どのくらい]

5　How long ＋ **does the pain** last?　どれくらいの間，痛みが続きますか．

6　How long ＋ have you had the pain?　（現在も痛みが続いている時）

7　How often ＋ do you have/experience the pain?　どのくらいの頻度で，痛みがありますか．

8　How often ＋ does it happen?　どのくらいの頻度で起こりますか．

練 習 このパターンで，ここまで話せる！　　　（解答は別冊）

42. 下痢をしますか．1日に何回くらい下痢がありましたか．
43. めまいが初めて起こったのはいつですか．
44. めまいが起こる前に，何か前兆はありますか．
45. 何か，痛みを改善したり，悪化したりするものはありますか．

内 科

Case 2-1　狭心症（54歳男性）

CD1 trk 3·7

Dr. Hello. How can I help you today?

Pt. I have chest pain.

Dr. Does it hurt now?（Are you having chest pain now?）

Pt. No, not at this moment.

Dr. When do you have pain?

Pt. Usually when I walk up stairs in the morning.

Dr. How long does it last?

Pt. It depends on the day. It generally lasts 3 to 4 minutes.

Dr. When you walk faster, does it get worse?

Pt. Yes, it does.

Dr. When did you experience this pain last?

Pt. About six months ago, I think. The pain is typically aggravated by cold weather.（The pain seems to get worse when it's cold.）

Dr. I see. Where exactly is the chest pain located?

Pt. The pain is in the middle and across the left side of my chest. When it gets worse, it seems to spread to my back.

Dr. I see. Let me take your blood pressure. 142 over 96, which is a bit high. Your pulse is 72.

Let me listen to your heart. Please pull up your shirt.

Pt. OK.

Dr. Your heart sounds are normal and without murmurs.

Let me do an ECG, chest X-ray, and blood tests. We can get the results of the ECG and chest X-ray soon. After receiving the blood test results, I will determine your treatment plan.

Dr. こんにちは．今日はどうされましたか．
Pt. 胸が痛みます．
Dr. 今現在も痛みますか．
Pt. 今は大丈夫です．
Dr. どういう時に痛みますか．
Pt. 朝，階段を上る時に痛くなります．
Dr. その痛みはどのくらいの時間続きますか．
Pt. その時によって違うのですが，ふつう，3〜4分ぐらいです．
Dr. 早く歩くと症状が強くなりますか．
Pt. はい．
Dr. いつぐらいからそういう症状があるのですか．
Pt. 半年ぐらい前からです．通常寒くなってきたらひどくなってきます．

Dr. わかりました．その胸の痛みはどの辺が痛みますか．
Pt. 胸の真ん中から左のほうです．強い時は背中も痛くなります．
Dr. そうですか．では，血圧を測りましょう．142/96 で少しあがっていますね．脈は72．では心臓の音を聞かせてください．シャツを上にあげていただけますか．
Pt. はい．
Dr. 心音に異常は認めません．心雑音も認めませんね．
それでは，心電図と胸のレントゲン写真，そして血液の検査をやりましょう．心電図とレントゲンはすぐ結果が出ます．血液検査の結果もみて，治療方針を決めましょう．

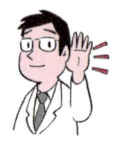

[Listening comprehension] (解答は別冊)

46. What is this patient's chief complaint?
47. Where is the pain located?

Easy Talk!　Speaking に便利な関係詞

Your blood pressure is 142 over 96, which is a bit high.　血圧は142/96で少し高いですね．

「それはね，それって，〜です」というように，which などの関係詞を用いて，関係詞の直前の名詞のさらに詳しい情報を付け加えます．

　　I can see a mass here which, I think, shows a tumor.
　　ここに腫瘤が見えます．それは(その腫瘤は)腫瘍と考えられます．

用語・用法研究：Which と that の使い分け

which は，その前の先行詞〔名詞〕が特定なものでなく，which 以下の付け足しの情報がなくても，文として成立する場合に用います．
that は，that 以下の説明がなければ先行詞〔名詞〕が特定できず，意味をなさない場合に用います．例えば，
a drug which was stored in the first aid box.　救急箱にあった薬
a drug that was stored in the first aid box.　救急箱にあった，その特定の薬

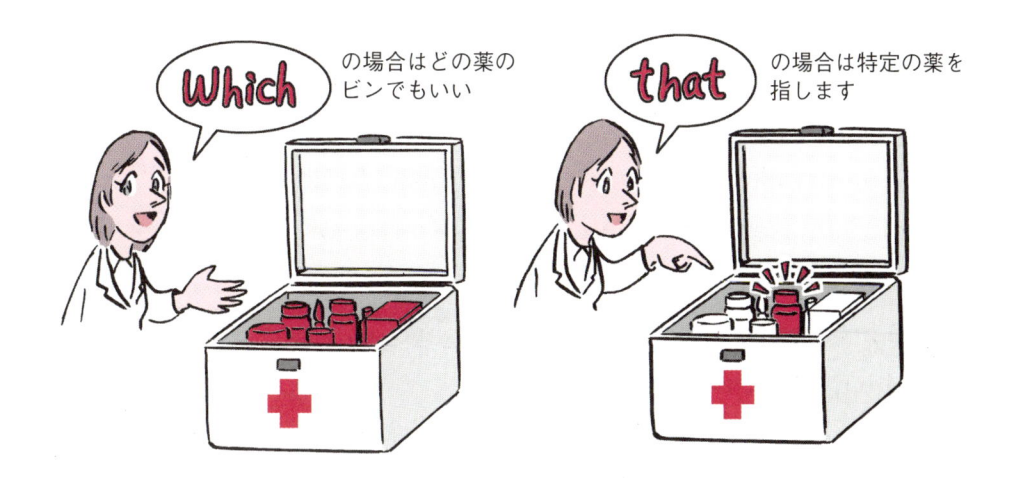

Which の場合はどの薬のビンでもいい

that の場合は特定の薬を指します

A drug which　A 薬　or　B 薬　or　C 薬　or　D 薬
A drug that　<u>A 薬</u>　B 薬　C 薬　D 薬

something や anything や everything や all などのあとに来る関係詞は that になります．
something that ～，anything that ～，everything that ～，all that などはフレーズとして使えるようにしましょう．
A doctor told us that we did <u>everything that</u> we could.「できるだけのことはしました」と医師は話した．

その他　the __est + 名 that　　先行詞が 人と物 の場合なども that を用います．
　　　（最上級の形容詞）

Case 2-2　狭心症(54歳男性)検査後

Dr. Sorry for keeping you waiting.

Pt. Doctor, what are the results?

Dr. The X-ray and ECG are normal.

Pt. I am happy to hear that. Does this mean I don't have any heart problems?

Dr. Not exactly. Even if no abnormality is detected, you may still have a potential heart problem. In your case, I think your chest pain is most likely caused by a heart problem, such as angina.

Pt. How is this treated?

Dr. First, I would like you to make appointments for three kinds of heart exams – cardiac ultrasonography, Holter ECG (a type of portable heart ECG with 24 hours recording) and exercise ECG.

Please make appointments later for a convenient time.

Pt. Sure, I will.

Dr. If you are diagnosed with angina through these examinations (Echo sound wave pictures, Holter and exercise ECG), you must have more thorough examinations, such as myocardial scintigraphy (a form of test used in nuclear medicine, in which radioisotopes are injected intravenously. Then gamma cameras capture and form images from the emitted ionizing radiation), CT (computed tomography) scan and catheter examination to assess coronary stenosis (abnormal narrowing of blood vessels surrounding the heart) and myocardial damage (heart muscle damage).

Based on the results of these detailed examinations, I'll determine the type of treatment you'll require. For example, whether you will need drugs or surgery.

Pt. It sounds like I have a serious disease.

Dr. No, don't worry so much. If you are treated properly at this early stage, you may be able to avoid serious heart problems in the future.

Pt. I see. I feel a bit relieved.

Dr. Do you know about a drug named Nitro?

Pt. I know it by name. My friends use it.

Dr. Nitro is a drug that reduces the burden on the heart by improving coronary blood flow, improving the supply of oxygen-rich blood to the heart muscle and reducing systemic vascular resistance.

It has few serious side effects. You may, however, experience temporary low blood pressure or headaches.

I'll prescribe the medication Nitro, today. Please carry it with you all the time, and if you have symptoms, please take it as directed.

If your symptoms resolve more quickly than usual, this typically means you are having real angina.

Dr. お待たせしました．
Pt. 先生，結果はどうですか．
Dr. レントゲンと心電図の結果は特に異常はありません．
Pt. ああ良かった．じゃあ，心臓の問題ではないのですね．
Dr. いいえ，所見がなくても心臓に病気がある場合もあります．ただ，あなたの場合は心臓疾患が原因の胸痛，例えば狭心症の可能性が高いと思います．
Pt. 治療はどうなりますか．
Dr. まず，これから3つの心臓の検査を予約していただこうと思います．それは，心臓の超音波検査，24時間心電図を記録するホルター心電図と，運動負荷心電図検査です．後で都合の良い日を予約してください．
Pt. 分かりました．
Dr. もし，これらの検査（エコー・ホルター・負荷心電図）で狭心症と診断された場合には，冠動脈の狭窄や心筋障害の評価をするため，心筋のシンチグラムやCT，カテーテル検査などさらに詳しい検査が必要になります．それらの結果をみて，薬物治療のみでよいか手術が必要なのかなど今後の治療方針を決めましょう．
Pt. なにか重い病気みたいですね．
Dr. いいえ，そんなに心配される必要はありません．もし，狭心症だとしても今の段階できちんと診断し治療をすれば，今後も心臓に重大な障害を残さずにすむと思いますよ．
Pt. わかりました．少し安心しました．
Dr. ニトロというお薬をご存知ですか．
Pt. はい，知人が使っているので，その名前だけは知っています．
Dr. ニトロは，心臓の血流を改善し，末梢血管の抵抗を下げて心臓にかかる負担を減らすお薬です．一時的に血圧が下がったり，頭痛が起こる場合はありますが，大きな副作用はありません．本日，ニトロを処方します．常に携帯していただき，胸痛発作が出た時に指示通り使ってください．ニトロを飲んで，症状がいつもよりスムースに改善するようなら，（本物の）狭心症の可能性がより高いということになります．

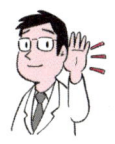

[Listening comprehension] (解答は別冊)

48. What is the most likely diagnosis?

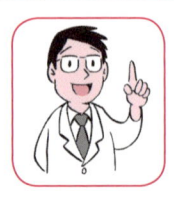

パターン6
～するために，治療・検査・手術が必要でしょう

1 You will need/require 検査・手術 to ～ （患者が主語の場合）
2 I will/am going to do 検査・手術 to ～ （医師が主語の場合）

例 You'll need to get a gastroscopy to ensure that you do not have a gastric ulcer.
　　胃潰瘍でないことを確認するために，胃カメラ検査をする必要があるでしょう．

文を分けて短文でも言うと
　⇒ I would like you to get a gastroscopy, so we can see if you have a gastric ulcer.
　　胃カメラ検査をしていただきます．そうすれば，潰瘍があるかみることができます．

●治療（検査・手術）などの目的を表す別の言い方を紹介します．

The purpose of the treatment is to ～　　治療（検査・手術）の目的は～です．

例 The purpose of diabetic treatment is to prevent secondary complications.
　　糖尿病の治療の目的は，続発する合併症を防ぐことです．

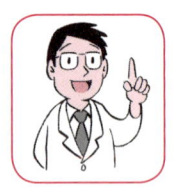

パターン7
検査の結果，（診断など）であることがわかりました

1 The test shows/demonstrates/reveals that ～
2 Looking at the results of the test, I think you have ～

Looking at the results of the test の代わりに，From the test results や After seeing the test results なども用いることができます．

例 Looking at the results of the test, you may have hepatitis.
　　検査の結果からすると，おそらく肝炎でしょう．

内　科

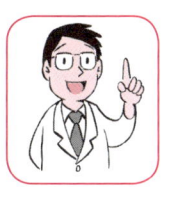

パターン8　〜のリスクについて説明する

1 There is a small risk of 〜/You may have a small risk of 〜
リスクが少しあります．

You have an increased risk of 〜　〜のリスクが増えています．

2 The benefits outweigh the risks of 〜　有益性が，リスクに勝っています．

例1　You have a small risk of bleeding.　出血の可能性が少しあります．

例2　The benefits of surgery outweigh the risks of possible complications or side effects associated with the surgery.
この手術は，手術によって引き起こされるかもしれない合併症または副作用のリスクより，手術による有益性のほうが大きいです．

A small risk of の代わりに，a small chance of, a slight possibility of に置き換えることができます．

あてはめましょう！

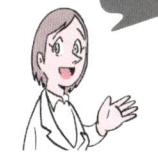

1　The symptoms 　示す　**a**　 you have 　診断名　**b**
この症状からみて，(診断名)でしょう．

2　　**c**　, I think you have diabetes.
〜から，糖尿病だと考えられます．

上記の **a, b, c** にそれぞれ以下の言葉をあてはめましょう．

a) suggest, demonstrate, indicate
b) a viral infection, kidney disease
c) Taking into account the results of the test 検査の結果を鑑みれば
　 Taking everything into consideration すべてのことを考慮すると
　 Based on this report この報告によると
　 Judging from your sugar levels 血中の糖の値から判断すると
　 On physical examination 診察では

33

パターン 9
安全であることを伝える

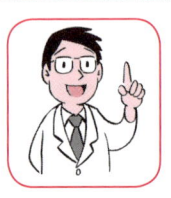

1 It shouldn't be a problem.
2 They are safe.
3 They are not dangerous.

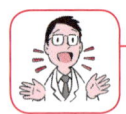

練習 このパターンでこれだけ話せる！　（解答は別冊）

49. 検査の結果，特に異常は認められませんでした．
50. HIV と HAV の迅速診断検査ができます．
51. 迅速インフルエンザ検査（RIDT）は，抗ウイルス薬を使用するかどうかを決定するために，症状が出現してから 48 時間以内に施行されるのが最も望ましい．
52. 結果は 10 分で出ます．
53. 入院が必要です．
54. 手術のため，一晩入院が必要です．
55. 心筋梗塞の可能性が最も高いでしょう．
56. 肺炎かどうかをみるために，レントゲン検査が必要です．
57. これらの検査の結果をみて，手術が必要かどうか決めましょう．
58. 検査の結果，腫瘍が充実性か，嚢胞性かどうかわかるでしょう．
59. 何もしない場合より，手術をすることにより脳卒中のリスクは低くなります．
60. 経過観察のため，4～6 時間病院にいてください．
61. 〔注射をする前にかける言葉〕ちくっとしますよ．

【ヒント】　充実性 solid

Case 3 糖尿病（45歳男性）

Dr. Hello. What is troubling you today?

Pt. I was told during a complete medical checkup that I have diabetes.

Dr. Let's see. HbA1c is 7.0 and urinalysis is positive for sugar(+1). There are otherwise no abnormalities. May I photocopy this report?

Pt. Yes.

Dr. Is this the first time you have been diagnosed with diabetes?

Pt. Yes. For the last few years I've been told at work check-ups and the like that I was on the verge of diabetes, but I was not told to get retested or anything.

Dr. I see. This new information indicates diabetes.

Pt. Will the medicine cure it?

Dr. It will improve. But, you must take medication for the rest of your life. Diabetes is not the kind of illness that is cured by medication.

Pt. It seems to be a complex disease.

Dr. Yes. If blood glucose levels rise abruptly, it can lead to sudden death. (sudden death can occur.) If diabetics fail to control their condition, they may suffer from various complications, leading to premature death. (that can even cause early death.) It is therefore important to maintain careful control. The main purpose of diabetic treatment is to prevent secondary complications or serious concurrent diseases, such as cerebral infarction (the ischemic kind of stroke) or myocardial infarction (a type of a heart attack).

Pt. I see. How do I control my conditon?

Dr. First, you must have your blood retested. As two months have passed since your last medical check-up, I would also like to see your HbA1c levels.

Pt. OK.

Dr. You must also follow a proper diet and exercise regimen. Concerning/ Regarding diet, the amount of calories you need depends on how much exercise you do on a daily basis.

Judging from your body composition (as determined by body mass index

(BMI)), you will need to limit your calories to about 2000 a day. A nutritionist will help explain this in greater detail.

Pt. I see.

Dr. Concerning exercise, aerobic exercises such as walking quickly, jogging, or swimming are particularly effective.

Pt. I see. Then, I will start with a morning walk.

Dr. It is important that you maintain your exercise. Make it a habit.

Pt. Yes, I will.

Dr. I'll take some blood for testing now. I will repeat this test in one month, so I'll be able to determine the effectiveness of your diet and exercise program. Taking these results into consideration, I'll then determine if you will require medication.

Pt. I see. Thank you.

Dr. こんにちは．今日はどうされましたか．
Pt. 人間ドックで糖尿病を指摘されました．
Dr. そうですね．
HbA1cが7.0ですね．あと，尿糖が（＋）〈ワンプラス〉，他にこれといった異常はありませんね．これをコピーをしてもいいですか．
Pt. はい．
Dr. 糖尿病を指摘されたのは今回が初めてですか．
Pt. はい．ここ数年，職場健診などで糖尿病のなりかけと言われたことはありますが，再検査などの指示はありませんでした．
Dr. そうですか．今回のデータからは，もう糖尿病ですね．
Pt. 薬を飲めば治りますか．
Dr. よくはなるでしょう．しかし，糖尿病は，薬で治るような病気ではなく，一生付き合っていかなければなりません．
Pt. めんどうですね．
Dr. ええ．血糖が極端に上がると急死することがあります．また，コントロールがよくないとさまざまな合併症を併発し，死に至るおそれもあるので，ご自身で自己管理をすることが大切です．糖尿病の治療の最大の目的は将来に起こる合併症や，脳梗塞・心筋梗塞などの重大な病気の併発を予防することなのです．
Pt. そうですか．実際にはどうしたらよいですか．
Dr. まず，血液の再検査を受けてください．健診からほぼ2ヵ月たっているので，HbA1c値を確認してみましょう．
Pt. はい．
Dr. 次に，食事療法と運動療法が必要になります．食事療法ですが，運動量にもよりますが，あなたの体格指数（BMI値）からは一日2000kcal程度に食事を制限する必要があると思います．そのやり方などは，詳しくは後ほど栄養士が説明いたします．
Pt. 了解しました．
Dr. 運動療法は，早足での散歩，ジョギング，水泳などの有酸素運動が特に有効です．
Pt. そうですか．とりあえず朝の散歩から始めてみます．
Dr. 継続が大切なので，慣れるまでは努力して続けてくださいね．
Pt. はい．
Dr. それではこれから採血をしましょう．また，次回1ヵ月後に検査をして，本日の結果と比べることで食事や運動の効果を決定しましょう．その状況で，お薬が必要かどうかを判断します．
Pt. わかりました．ありがとうございました．

内　科

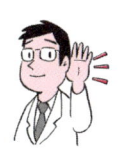

Listening comprehension （解答は別冊）

62. What determined this patient's diagnosis?

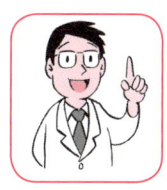

パターン 10
1 病気／症状は〜が原因でしょう
2 〜が，病気／症状の原因でしょう

1 病気・症状 is caused by 原因

Is caused by の代わりに，arises from/comes from/is due to なども使います．

2 原因 is causing 病気・症状

is causing の代わりに
　　is responsible for/is the cause of/
　　is linked to 〜/is related to 〜　　〜に関与しています．
なども使えます．

例1　The symptoms may be caused by a diseased tooth.
　　その症状は，虫歯が原因の可能性があります．
例2　Is my bad tooth causing this inflammation?
　　虫歯が炎症をひきおこしているのですか．

Case 4-1　頸部リンパ節腫脹（28歳女性）

Dr. Hello. What brings you in today?
Pt. My neck's been swollen for about a week.
Dr. Which part of your neck?
Pt. Here.
〔*The patient points to the bottom left side of the neck.*〕
Dr. 〔*Palpating*〕 Is this where the pain is?
Pt. Ouch...
Dr. Oh, sorry. Does it hurt, when I touch this?
Pt. Yes. The swelling has gotten bigger and the pain has gotten worse since yesterday.
Dr. I see. Do you have a fever?
Pt. No, I don't think so.
Dr. Let me take your temperature.
Ns. Please put this thermometer under your arm.
Pt. Sure.
Dr. I'd like to ask some questions while your temperature is being taken.
　　Do you have any cold-like symptoms, such as a sore throat or a runny nose?
Pt. No, I don't think I have a cold.
Dr. Okay. Let me take a look at your throat.
Pt. Sure.
Dr. Open your mouth wide and say "ahh" loudly.
Pt. "Ahh..."
Dr. Okay, that's it.
Ns. Please give me the thermometer. It's 37.2.
Dr. You have a low grade fever. You don't seem to have any serious problems with your throat. Do you have a decayed tooth (dental caries)?
Pt. I may. I sometimes feel pain in my back tooth. I should consult a dentist.
Dr. Yes, the symptoms may arise from a diseased tooth or inflamed gums.

Pt. Do you think my bad tooth is causing this?

Dr. I cannot say yes with 100% certainty. However, there is a possibility of that. Your neck pain may be caused by swelling of lymph nodes, probably due to a bacterial infection. If you have swelling and pain on one side of the neck without any other throat problems, the condition (cervical lymphadenitis) is frequently associated with a decayed tooth or gum disease (periodontal disease).

Pt. I see. I'll go to see a dentist.

Dr. When will you go?

Pt. My dentist is by advance appointment, so I will make an appointment straight away.

Dr. OK, I will give you three days of antibiotics and a painkiller for provisional treatment. Please consult a dentist as soon as possible.

Dr. 今日はどうされましたか.
Pt. 1週間ぐらい前から、頸が腫れているのです.
Dr. 頸のどこですか.
Pt. ここの部分です〔左の顎の付け根のやや下を指す〕
Dr. 〔触診をしながら〕これですね.
Pt. あいたたた・・・.
Dr. あ、ごめんなさい. 触るといたみますか.
Pt. ええ、昨日ぐらいから腫れがひどくなって、痛みも強くなりました.
Dr. 熱がありますか.
Pt. 自分では感じませんが・・.
Dr. では、熱を測ってみましょう.
Ns. これ(体温計)をわきの下に挟んでください.
Pt. はい.
Dr. 測りながらお聞きしますが、喉の痛みや、鼻水など、かぜの症状はありませんか.
Pt. いいえ、かぜをひいたと言う感じはしません.
Dr. そうですか. 一応、喉を見せてください.
Pt. はい.
Dr. では、口をあけて、アーと声を出してください.
Pt. アー.
Dr. はい、いいですよ.

Ns. それでは、体温計をください. 37.2度ですね.
Dr. 熱は微熱ですね. 喉はそんなに悪くありません. 虫歯はありますか.
Pt. 虫歯があるかもしれません. 時々奥歯が痛む感じもあって歯医者さんに行かなければと思っていました.
Dr. そうですね. 頸の症状は虫歯か、歯肉の炎症から来ているかもしれませんね.
Pt. 虫歯が原因ですか.
Dr. 100%断定はできませんが、その可能性がありますね. 頸のリンパ腺が腫れて痛みが出ているのですが、多分細菌感染によるものと思います.
痛みを伴って片方だけ腫れていて、喉の所見が問題ない場合は、歯から来ていることが多いのですよ.
Pt. そうですか. では、歯医者さんに行ってきます.
Dr. いつ行かれますか.
Pt. 私のかかりつけの歯医者さんは、予約制ですから、すぐに予約を入れてみます.
Dr. そうですか. それではとりあえず、痛み止めと抗菌剤を3日分出しておきますので、なるべく早く、診てもらうようにしてくださいね.

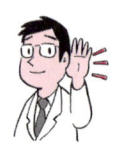

Listening comprehension

(解答は別冊)

63. What are the patient's complaints? Please choose the correct ones.
    A. neck pain   B. high fever   C. leg swelling
    D. neck swelling   E cold-like symptoms

Case 4-2　頸部リンパ節腫脹（28歳女性）：歯科受診

Dentist(Dr.)　Hello. I hear you have pain in your lower left back tooth. Have you taken the medicine prescribed by your physician?

Pt.　Yes, I have and the pain goes away.

Dr.　Alright. If the pain goes away, please stop taking the pain killers. Have you ever had these symptoms before?

Pt.　No. This is the first time.

Dr.　May I take a look inside your mouth?

Your wisdom tooth is now coming out, so this could be the cause of the pain. But you also have dental caries near the wisdom tooth in question. This may also be responsible for the pain.

Let me take an X-ray to examine this more closely.

〔*After taking the X-ray*〕

Dr.　The X-ray shows inflammation around your wisdom tooth. Usually, the affected tooth should be extracted. But in your case, the inflammation (gingivitis) is already subsided and not recurred, so I recommend teeth cleaning and follow-up check-ups.

Pt.　I see.

Dr.　I would like to treat the dental cavities. Nerves within your chin may be responsible for the pain you've been experiencing.

Pt.　How long will the treatment take to complete?

Dr.　If the decay hasn't reached the tooth nerve, you will probably require only two or three sessions. If it has progressed into the tooth nerve, you may have to come in for up to ten sessions.

内 科

It depends on your condition moving forward, so it is difficult to say.

Dr. こんにちは，本日は左下の奥歯が痛むとのことですが，内科で処方されたお薬を飲まれましたか．
Pt. はい，今は痛みがおさまりました．
Dr. そうですか．痛みがおさまったならば，痛み止めの服用は中止してください．今までも，このような症状はありましたか．
Pt. 初めてです．
Dr. お口の中を見せてください．
親知らずが崩出しかけているため，これが原因かと考えられますが，手前にも虫歯があるため，これが原因の可能性もあります．レントゲンで詳しく調べてみましょう．
〔レントゲンのあとで〕
Dr. 今，とったレントゲンですが，やはり親知らずのあたりが炎症を起こしています．
根本的な解決策としては，親知らずを抜いてしまうことになりますが，歯肉炎を繰り返しているわけでなければ，今回は症状もおさまっていることですし，クリーニングをして経過観察という方法も良いかと思います．
Pt. わかりました．
Dr. 虫歯があるので，治療をしていきましょう．顎の中の神経が，痛みの原因であることも考えられます．
Pt. 治療にはどのくらいの期間がかかりますか．
Dr. 虫歯が神経まで及んでいない場合は，2，3回で終わります．人によって様々であるため，はっきりと申し上げにくいのですが，神経までいっていた場合，10回位は通う事になると思います．

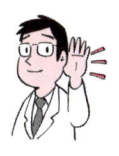

[Listening comprehension]　　　　　　　　　　（解答は別冊）

64. What is the most likely diagnosis?

🖈 **用語・用法の研究**

"session"は治療の回数を意味し，"visit"は来院の回数を意味します．ですから理論上は1回の来院時に2回の治療を受けることもあるわけですが，実際には1回の来院では1回の治療です．

💬 **coffee break**

主に，内科からリンパ腫脹等で歯科治療を依頼される時は，奥歯（臼歯部）molars の虫歯か，親知らずの影響で顎の付け根の部分が腫れていると考えられる場合が多いです．また，歯科では，内科等のリスク患者に関しては，ほとんどの場合，ケースバイケースで内科の医師と随時連絡を取りながら治療を行ってます．

▶歯科でよく用いる会話例

■受付にて保険に関する質問
Will the insurance pay for it? The insurance won't pay for it. 保険が使えますか．保険は使えません．
(= Is it covered by my insurance? It is not covered by the insurance.)
The treatment will be at your own expense. 自費での治療になります．

■痛みに関する質問
Which tooth aches? This (upper) tooth aches. どの歯が痛みますか．この(上の)歯が痛いです．
My lower front (back) tooth aches. 下の前歯(奥歯)が痛みます．
When did it start hurting? いつ痛み始めましたか．
Does it hurt when you eat something cold or hot? 冷たいものや温かいものにしみますか．
Does it hurt when you chew? 噛むと痛みますか．

■歯の状態の説明
Food often gets stuck in this part. 食物がよくこの部分に詰ります．
Pus has built up at the end of the root. 歯根部に膿がたまっています．
There's something not right about your bite. 少し噛み合わせが悪いです．

The nerve of the tooth is also damaged. 神経まで損傷しています．
The cavity has reached the tooth's nerve. 虫歯は歯の神経まで進んでいます．
You have gingivitis (periodontitis) (pyorthea). あなたは，歯肉炎(歯周病)(歯槽膿漏)があります．
Your teeth are covered with plaque. あなたの歯は歯垢がついています．
It has festered. 化膿しています．
The gums around the wisdom tooth are swollen and contain pus. 親知らずの周辺の歯ぐきは，膨れて膿を持っています．

■治療方法の説明
We should remove your tartar. 歯石を取ったほうが良いでしょう．
We will use an ultrasonic scaler 超音波スケーラーを使います．
I will use filling material that is covered by the insurance. 保険でできる材料で歯に詰めます．
We will have to treat the root canal. 根管治療をしなければなりません
I will check your bite. 噛み合わせをみます．
I will extract the tooth's nerve. 歯の神経を取ります．
I extracted the nerve from the tooth. 歯の神経を取りました．
I will clean and treat the inside of your root canal. 根管の中をきれいにします．
I've finished the root canal treatment, so I will fill the cavity now. 根管治療が終わりましたので，充填剤を詰めます．
I will cut the gum to drain the pus. 歯肉を切って膿を出します．
Your tooth is out now, so please bite down strongly on this gauze. 歯を抜きました．このガーゼを強く噛んでください．
Please bite on this gauze for about 20 minutes, until the bleeding stops. 出血が止まるまで，約20分間このガーゼを噛んでください．
Please place your chin on this rest. 顎をこの台の上に置いてください．
Please rinse your mouth. 口をすすいでください．
Please bite on this a few times. これを数回噛んでください．

If it hurts, please raise your left hand. 痛い時は，左手を上げてください.

■注射・麻酔
I am going to inject the anesthetic, so please don't move. 動かないで，麻酔薬を注射します.
I will use an inhalable sedative. 吸入麻酔します.
Please inhale through your nose. 鼻から吸入してください.
The numbness will go away after about two to three hours. 麻酔は，約2～3時間効いています.
Please eat after the numbness passes. 麻酔が覚めた後で，食べてください.
Your tongue, cheeks, and lips are numb, so please try not to bite them while eating. 麻酔しているので食べる時，舌，頬や口唇を噛まないようにしてください.

■指示
Please use dental floss to clean between your teeth. 歯と歯の間をきれいにするには糸ようじを使ってください.
Please massage your gums. 歯肉をマッサージしてください.
Please come to have your tartar removed every 6 months. 6ヵ月ごとに歯石を取りに来てください.

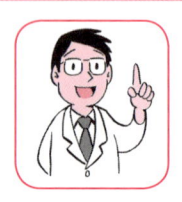

パターン 11
指示 1
〜をとってください，〜を避けてください，薬などを出しましょう

1. Please take 〜
2. Please refrain from/avoid/stop 〜
3. I am going to 〜/I will give you 〜

例 1　Please make sure you take/receive adequate rest　必ず，休養を十分にとってください．
　　　You may also consider a vitamin supplement.　ビタミン剤をとってもいいでしょう．

例 2　Please refrain from/avoid excess salt.　塩分は控えてください．

例 3　I am going to/am giving you antibiotics. Please take two pills four times a day.
　　　抗生剤を出しますので，1回2錠，1日4回お飲みください．

words and expressions
bid：1日2回　tid：1日3回　q.i.d：1日4回
「10mg/kg bid」の場合，10mg/kg を1日2回に分けて投与（総量 10mg/kg/day）
*（注：今後の記載は，●mg/kg/回×●回/日が基本処方となります）

■その他：再診の指示例

4. Please come back for a check-up a week from now.
　一週間後に様子をみせてください．

5. Should any emergency scenario arise, please return promptly to the clinic. (If there are any problems, please come back here as soon as possible.)
　病状が急変したらすぐ来てください（もし何かあったら，できるだけ早く来てください）．

内 科

あてはめましょう！

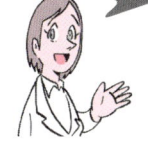

次の枠内に (a)(b) の用語をあてはめて，症状を尋ねてください．

(a) 〜もとりましょう　**You may also consider** ☐

(b) 〜を避けてください　**Please avoid** ☐

(a) iron supplements 鉄剤，calcium supplements カルシウム剤，
enough plant protein 十分な植物性タンパク質，enough sleep 十分な睡眠

(b) fatty foods 油っこい食品，spicy foods 刺激物，direct sunlight 直射日光，strenuous exercise 激しい運動，alcohol in excess 飲みすぎ，smoking 喫煙

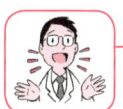

練習 このパターンでこれだけ話せる！ （解答は別冊）

65. 十分な水分をお取りください．
66. 適度な運動をしてください．
67. 指示通り，これらの薬をお飲みください．
68. 1カプセルずつお飲みください．
69. 必要に応じて，軟膏，クリームをお使いください．
70. 1日2錠ずつ1日3回を1週間お飲みください．
71. 再診の予約をお取りください．

📌 Common Contraction

Does she~?	Du シッ
Do you~?	ジュ
Did you~?	ディッ　ジャ
What do you~?	**wa** チャ
What did you~?	**wa** ジャ
What are you~?	**wa** チャ
Why do you~?	**why** ジュ
Why did you~?	**why** ジャ
Are you~?	ヤ
going to	ゴナ
got to	ゴタァ / ゴル
have to	ハ f タ
want to	**wo** ナ
would not have	**wu**dn ナ
should not have	シュ dn ナ
Let me	**l** ミー

45

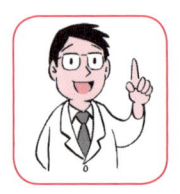

パターン 12
指示 2
〜するとよいでしょう．ぜひ〜しましょう

1 It might be better/a good idea to 〜

"might"の代わりに"would"を用いるともう少し強い言い方になります．
might be better の代わりに，is necessary, is important, is essential, is vital などに置き換えるとさらに強い指示になります．

2 It is (very) important/crucial that you (should) ＋原型動詞

(1 の表現に比べ少し formal な言い方になります)

3 I (strongly) recommend/suggest that you (should) ＋原型動詞

that 節の主語 (you) の後は should ＋原型動詞がきます．should を省くこともできます．

例 1 It might be better to check the blood vessels in your brain.
　　　脳の血管を調べたほうがいいでしょう．

例 2 It is important for your health that your gum disease be controlled.
　　　歯周病をコントロールすることは，体全体の健康に大切なことです．

例 3 I recommend that you have a head MRI.　頭の MRI を受けましょう．

● I would like you to 〜/I want to ask you to 〜してくださいね．という構文で簡単に伝えることもできます．

例　I would like you to take a blood test.
　　血液検査を受けてください．

● 患者を主語にして，You need to 〜, You should 〜, You (really) must 〜などさらに簡単に言うこともできます．

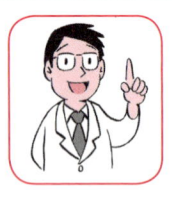

パターン 13
紹介状を書く

I'll write a referral letter for you to a specialist
　　　　＋ so please go to the hospital ＋ as soon as possible (ASAP)

専門医に紹介状を書いておきますから，なるべく早く，病院へ行ってください．

Case 5　高血圧症（66 歳女性）

Pt. While bending over for gardening a couple of days ago, I felt a bit faint and the back of my head felt heavy. I thought it might be due to stiff shoulders, but because I felt a bit dizzy, I took my blood pressure just in case, and it was 180 over 110. My blood pressure has been normal up to now, and they've never mentioned anything unusual in my blood tests at my medical check-ups.

Dr. Have you been under stress recently? Do you drink or smoke a lot?

Pt. Well, now you mention it, my brother was admitted to the hospital recently. I smoke 40 (2 packs) a day. I used to drink 2 or 3, small cans of beer a day, but I stopped drinking when this started.

Dr. Your brother's hospitalization might be the trigger for this. Now I'll examine you.

〔After performing X-ray, ECG, and US〕

Dr. Please stop smoking and drinking for a while and take things easy at home. Could you make a note of your blood pressure when you get up and before you go to bed? Since the pressure has gone up abruptly, I think it might be better to check the blood vessels in your brain.
I recommend that you have a head MRI scan, and an MRA scan to visualize the blood vessels.

Pt. I see. Do these tests hurt?

Dr. No, they don't hurt, but they can be hard for people with claustrophobia. Also, people with pacemakers shouldn't take them. You also need to see an opthalmologist to check whether there is anything wrong with the blood vessels in the back of your eye. I'll write you a referral letter. Because your symptoms are severe, I'll start off with a low dose of anti-hypertensive drugs. I'll also give you a small dose of tranquilizers, so please be careful while driving. If you can't sleep well, take a low dose of sleeping pills. I want to keep an eye on the changes in your blood pressure for a while, so please come back frequently.

Pt. 2～3日前から花の手入れなどで下を向いたらくらっとして後頭部が重い感じがしました．肩こりのためと思いました．少し，フラフラするので，念のため血圧を測ったら180/110もありました．いままで血圧は異常がなかったし，健診で，血液検査にも異常を言われたことはありません．

Dr. 最近何かストレスになるようなことはありませんでしたか．お酒やタバコの量が多くはないですか．

Pt. そういえば，最近弟が入院しました．タバコは1日に40本吸います．ビールは350ml缶を2～3本飲んでいましたが，このようになってからは飲んでいません．

Dr. ご兄弟の入院がきっかけかもしれませんね．それでは診察しましょう．
〔胸部レントゲン検査，心電図や心エコーを試行した後〕

Dr. しばらく酒もタバコもやめて，ゆったり家ですごしてください．自宅での血圧を起床時と寝る前，記録してもらえますか．また，急に血圧が高くなって来ているので，脳血管についても調べたほうがいいかと思います．頭のMRIと脳の血管を描き出すMRAという検査を受けていただけますか．

Pt. わかりました．その検査は痛いですか．

Dr. 痛い検査ではありませんが，閉所恐怖症の方は難しい場合があります．また，ペースメーカーを入れている方はできません．
また，眼底血管に異常があるかどうか，眼科を受診していただけますか．紹介状を書いておきます．症状が強いので，降圧剤を少量から開始します．精神安定剤も少量投与しますので，車の運転には注意してください．夜眠れないようなら，睡眠剤を少し飲んでください．しばらく，血圧の推移をみたいので，頻回に受診してください

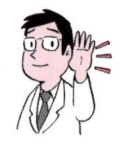

Listening comprehension

（解答は別冊）

72. What is the most likely diagnosis?

Easy talk! "so"は，日本語の「そうだから・それで」とほぼ同じような感じで用いることができ，診療でも広く活用できます（⇒長い説明は，短文に切り接続詞を活用）．

PART 1

小児科

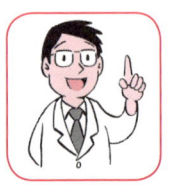

パターン 1
子供の症状を家族に尋ねる
症状があったようですか

1 Does your son/daughter have 症状 ?

2 Have you noticed 症状 ?

例1 Does your son have a cough with wheezing while sleeping?
　　息子さんは，寝ている間，喘鳴を伴って咳をしていましたか．

例2 Have you noticed any blood in his stool?
　　便に血が混ざっていることに気がつきましたか．

Easy talk !

[部品交換] 部品交換つまり，単語やフレーズを部分的に交換することで会話を広げることができます．

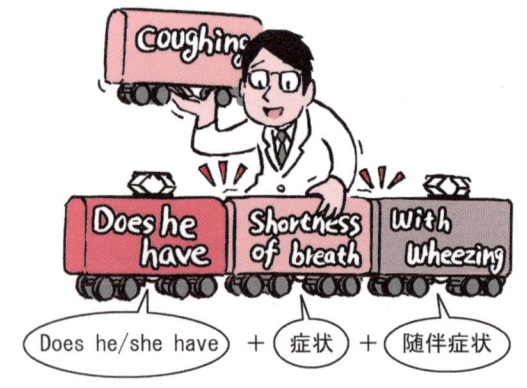

Does he/she have ＋ 症状 ＋ 随伴症状

Real English のコツ：部品交換も，同じような状況で，なるべくネイティブスピーカーの表現を，そのまま使いましょう．

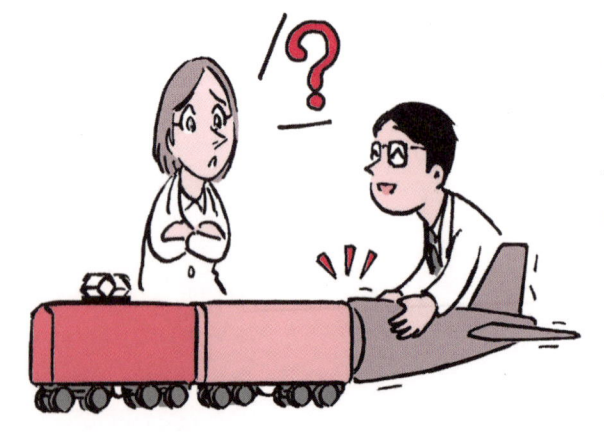

日本語をそのまま英訳しても？？？
例：「つまらないものですが，どうぞ.」という日本語をそのまま英訳し，"This is a trivial gift, but please accept it." と言っても，「どうして，つまらないものをわざわざプレゼントするのだろう．はてな？？」となり，意味が通じません．

小児科

Easy talk！
［主文導入部追加］

英文はしばしば，「～に気がつきましたか．～しているようですか．」は会話の最初に付け足し，そのあとに，主文が続きます．

お子さんがゼーゼー言いながら息切れをしていたことがありますか．
Have you noticed whether he has shortness of breath with wheezing?

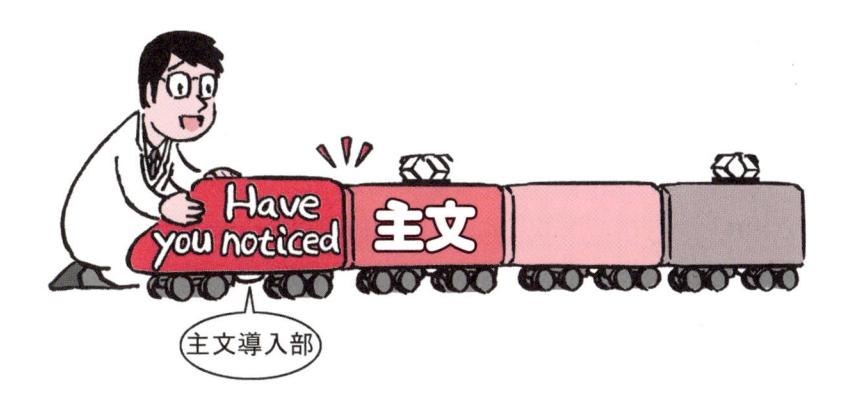

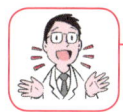

主文導入部

練習　このパターンでこれだけ話せる！　　（解答は別冊）

〔母親（父親）に子どもの様子を尋ねてみましょう〕
73. 痛みは消えたようですか．
74. いつごろ，痛いといいましたか．
75. どのような時，良くなったり，ひどくなったりしているようですか．
76. 痛みは出てきたり，治まったりするようですか．
77. 痛みはずっと続いているようですか，それとも痛くなったりおさまったりするようですか．
78. 便に血が混じっていたのに気がつきましたか．
79. あなたのお子様が難聴になったのにいつ気がつきましたか．

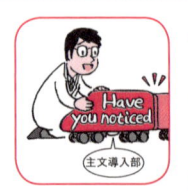

パターン2
診断・検査・指示などによく用いる主文導入部のフレーズ（1）

主文の前に付け足すフレーズとして言い慣れておきましょう．（注：文法的な構文は異なるものも含まれます．和訳は，会話用にできるだけ英語の語順で訳しています．）

I think ＋（**that**）＋ he has acute pneumonia.
考えますが，お子さんは急性肺炎だと．

I don't think ＋（**that**）＋ she has exanthema subitum.
考えませんが，お子さんは，突発疹であるとは．

I suspect ＋（**that**）＋ your baby has Kawasaki disease.
疑いですが，お子さんは川崎病でしょう．

I am afraid ＋（**that**）＋ he has leukemia.
残念ですが，お子さんは白血病です．

I recommend ＋（**that**）＋ you take her to a specialist as soon as possible.
是非，できるだけ早く専門医にみてもらってください．

It's most likely ＋（**that**）＋ he has group A streptococcal infection.
最も可能性が高いのは，お子さんはA群溶連菌症です．

It seems ＋（**that**）＋ she has acute pyelonephritis.
おそらく，お子さんは急性腎盂炎でしょう．

It is important ＋（**that**）＋ your son has allergy tests.
大切なことは，お子さんがアレルギー検査を受けることです．

The point is they're not getting the proper medical treatment. 要は，彼らが適切な治療を受けていないことです．「要点は〜」「要は〜」「大切なことは〜」などの意味のフレーズには The point is 〜/Thing is 〜（very casual expression）/The important thing is 〜などもよく用いられます．

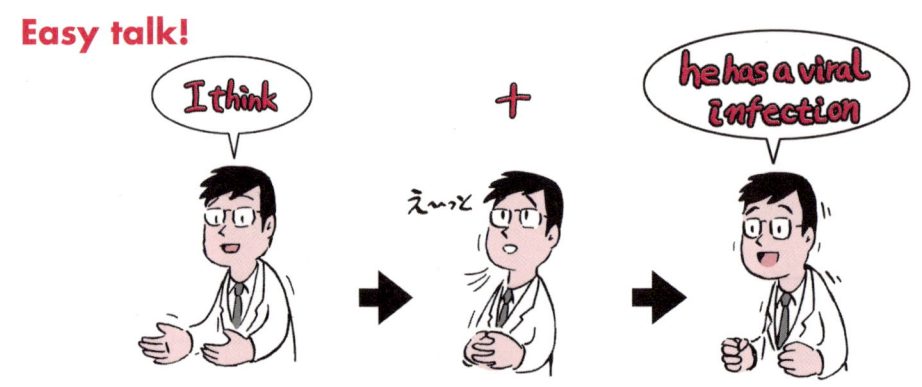

Easy talk!

ここで短い息つぎをしてもいいですね．

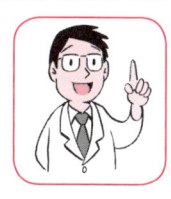

小児科

パターン3
主文導入部のフレーズ(2)

1 **I am pleased to say** ＋（**that**）＋ we can fix it for him.
   いいお知らせですが，息子さんを治すことができます．
2 **We can say** ＋（**that**）＋ we can make things a lot better.
   お話しできることは，ずっと良くなるということです．
3 **This means** ＋（**that**）＋ he doesn't need an operation.
   つまり，お子様は手術の必要がありません．
4 **It appears** ＋（**to me**）（**that**）＋ the mass is a bit enlarged.
   見たところ，腫瘍は少し大きくなっているようです．

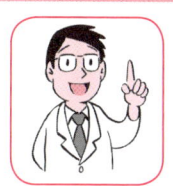

パターン4
症状が認められますか

Is 　症　状　 present/observed?

例　Is enteritis present/observed?
　　腸炎が認められますか．

※医師間やプレゼンなどで用いるややフォーマルな表現

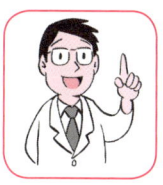

パターン5
随伴症状を別の言い方で尋ねる

Is 　症　状　 accompanied by 　随伴症状　 ?

例　Is abdominal pain accompanied by diarrhea or fever?
　　腹痛に下痢または熱が伴っていますか．

Does 　症　状　 come with 　随伴症状　 ? または，
Does he have 　症　状　 and 　随伴症状　 ? などもいえます．

53

📌 メディカルコーナー　診察時，一度に多くの症状の有無について尋ねる場合

多くの症状の有無を一度に尋ねるかわりに，下記⇒のように，症状を順に尋ねましょう．

例　Do you have any pain, fever or nausea and vomiting?
　　　痛みあるいは熱，吐き気と嘔吐はありますか．

⇒1　Do you have any pain?　痛みはありますか．
　2　How about a fever?　熱はいかがですか．
　3　Any nausea or vomiting?　吐き気と嘔吐は？

あてはめましょう！

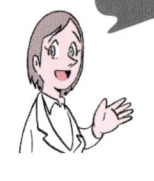

次の枠内に下記の (a) (b) の用語をそれぞれあてはめて，症状を尋ねてください．

(a)　Does your son have ⬜ ?
(b)　Have you noticed whether/if he has ⬜ ?

(a)　ear pain 耳の痛み，allergies アレルギー，tinnitus（ringing in the ear）耳鳴り
(b)　coughing 咳，abdominal pain 腹痛，diarrhea（loose stools）下痢，tarry stools タール便，constipation 便秘，jaundice 黄疸，pelvic pain 骨盤痛，appetite changes 食欲の変化，ear discharge 耳だれ，foot pain 足の痛み

あてはめましょう！

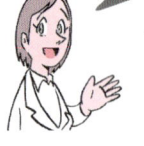

次の枠内に下記 (a) (b) の用語をそれぞれあてはめて症状を尋ねてください．

(a)　Is ⬜ present?
(b)　Is ⬜ observed?

(a)　ringing in the ear（tinnitus 耳鳴り），sore throat のどの痛み，hearing loss 聴力損失，an inguinal mass 鼠径部腫瘤，parotid gland swelling 耳下腺の腫れ
(b)　nausea 吐き気，vomiting 嘔吐，rash（exanthema）発疹，eczema 湿疹

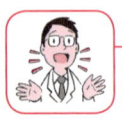

練習　このパターンでこれだけ話せる！　（解答は別冊）

80. お嬢さんは，3日間熱がありましたか．
81. 下痢以外に何か症状がありますか．
82. お子様は，犬が吠えるような（オットセイが鳴くような）咳をしますか．
83. 呼吸障害を伴って咳がありますか．
84. 腹痛に，悪心，嘔吐，下痢，便秘を伴っていますか．
85. けいれんに，高熱，意識障害を伴っていますか．

Case 6-1　腸重積症（生後 11 ヵ月男児）

Dr. Hello, how is your son feeling today?

Patient's mother. He's been in a terrible mood since this morning and has kept crying furiously/so hard about every 15 minutes. He also vomited.

Dr. Could you tell me what time this started? And, how often has he vomited?

M. This began around 6:30 AM, and he vomited three times. Up to that point, he had been fine and had drunk his milk well.

Dr. Let me examine him. He doesn't seem to have a fever, but he appears pale.

M. Yes, he looks paler than usual.

Dr. His breath sounds are clear to auscultation, but his throat is slightly red. Have you noticed any cold symptoms?

M. He's had cold-like symptoms and minor diarrhea for the past 2 to 3 days.

Dr. Ok. Let us put him on the bed.
〔*After examination.*〕His abdomen is bloated. I can feel a mass on his right upper abdomen. When I press there, he cries intensely. Have you noticed any blood in his stool?

M. No, I hadn't noticed any blood in his stool before last night. Since then, he hasn't passed any stool at all.

Dr. こんにちは．お子様はどうされましたか．
Patient's mother.（母）　朝から機嫌が非常に悪くて，15分おき位に激しく泣いています．嘔吐もみられます．
Dr. 何時ごろから始まりましたか．そして何回吐きましたか．
M.（母）　今朝の6時30分ごろからで嘔吐は3回です．それまでは元気にミルクを飲んでいました．
Dr. それでは診察してみましょう．熱はないようですが，顔色が悪いですね．
M.（母）　はい，いつもより青白いと思います．

Dr. 胸の聴診では異常はないようですが，のどが少し赤いようです．かぜ症状はありませんでしたか．
M.（母）　2〜3日前からかぜ気味で，少し下痢がありました．
Dr. わかりました．それではベッドにあおむけに寝かせてください．〔診察後〕お腹が張っていますね．右上腹部に腫瘤をふれます．そこを押さえると，激しく泣きますね．血便はみられませんでしたか．
M.（母）　昨夜までの便に血は混じっていませんでしたが，それ以降は便は出ていません．

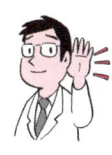

Listening comprehension
（解答は別冊）

86. What is the patient's chief complaint?

Case 6-2　腸重積症（生後11ヵ月男児）

Dr. OK, I'll administer a glycerin enema (GE) to see if there is blood in the stool.

〔*Following the GE.*〕I see blood in his stool. Given his symptoms and the abdominal mass, I suspect he has an intussusception. I'll perform an ultrasonic test to be sure of this.

〔*After the ultrasonic test.*〕As the ultrasound shows a tumor mass, an intussusception is likely. Some mesenteric lymph nodes are swollen, but intestinal obstruction looks mild.

M. How is this treated?

Dr. I'll try a hydrostatic enema reduction now. Is that ok with you? If we are not able to fix it with this procedure, he may need surgical care/surgery.

〔*Following the reduction during us exam.*〕

Dr. Fortunately, his intussusception was successfully reduced hydrostatically.

M. Thank you very much.

Dr. He needs to remain overnight in the hospital to receive IV fluids. Intussusceptions relapse in about 5 to 10% of cases. It's rare that there are other organic diseases that may be responsible for the intussusception.（Very occasionally, other organic disease can cause the intussusceptions.）A nurse will be happy to explain the procedure for his admission.

Dr. わかりました．それでは，血が便に混じっているかどうかを見るために，浣腸してみましょう．
〔浣腸後〕
血便がみられますね．症状と腹部の腫瘤から，腸重積症の可能性が大きいようです．確認するために超音波検査を施行してみましょう．
〔超音波検査後〕
超音波検査にても腫瘤がみられ，腸重積症でしょう．腸間膜のリンパ節も腫れているようですが，腸閉塞は軽度と考えられます．

M.（母）　治療はどうなりますでしょうか．

Dr. これから高圧注腸整復術を試みましょう．それでは，これから整復してみますが，よろしいでしょうか．
もしこれで整復できなければ，手術が必要になります．
〔超音波検査下整復後〕

Dr. お母さんよかったですね．無事に高圧注腸にて整復することができました．

M.（母）　ありがとうございました．

Dr. 一晩入院して点滴していただきます．腸重積症は，5～10％位に再発する事があります．まれですが，腸重積症をひきおこす別の腸の器質的疾患があることもあります．では，看護師が入院の手続きをいたします．

小児科

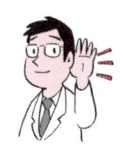

Listening comprehension （解答は別冊）

87. What is the most likely diagnosis?

> **Coffee Break**　腸重積症の原因
>
> 原因不明とされているが，先行することの多いウイルスや細菌の感染による腸間膜リンパ節腫大やパイエル板肥厚などの関与が示唆されている．器質的原因としては，Meckel憩室，ポリープ，腸管重複症，悪性リンパ腫などが約5％にみられる．

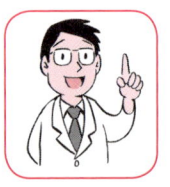

パターン6
診察時の会話

1. Now I'll examine 体の部位　それでは～をみましょう．
   examine の代わりに take a look at に置き換えることもできます．
   また，I'll examine を I'm going to examine ともいえます．

●聴力を調べる

2. I'm going to check your hearing. I'll snap my fingers by your ear, so please tell me which side you hear the sound.
   耳の聞こえ具合を調べましょう．耳のそばで指を鳴らしますから，どちら側で音が聞こえるかを知らせてくださいね．

3. Does anyone in your family (the day nursery/kindergarten/school) have similar symptoms?
   ご家族(保育園/幼稚園/学校)で同じような症状の人はいますか．

4. Good boy/girl. Now it's over.　いい子ね．さあ，終わりましたよ．

あてはめましょう！

枠内に下記の用語をあてはめましょう．

I'll/am going to ☐

tap on your chest. 胸をトントンしますよ．　tap on your tummy. お腹をトントンしますよ．
listen to your heart. 心臓の音を聞きますよ．　listen to your lungs. 胸の音を聞きますよ．
press on your belly. お腹を押さえますよ．

小児科

Case 7-1 インフルエンザ（7歳女児） *trk 13-17*

Dr. Good morning. What seems to be the problem with your daughter today?

M. My daughter ran a high fever all of a sudden, so I got worried about her and brought her to see you, doctor.

Dr. Since when has she had it and what was her body temperature?

M. She has had a high fever since yesterday evening. It increased to 39.4 .

Dr. Does she have any other symptoms?

M. She had a cough and pain in her head, arms, and legs. She also seems to have abdominal pain, but, she doesn't have any diarrhea or vomiting. She just appears lethargic.

Dr. Ok, I'll examine her now. Now, Jane, let me listen to your lungs. Please lift up your shirt and expose your chest. Please turn around and let me take a look at your back. I think that her lung sounds are clear. Now, let me take a look at your ears. She doesn't seem to have otitis media. Please open your mouth nice and wide, and say 'ah'. Her throat seems to be a bit injected （red）. Is there anyone around her who has similar symptoms?

M. I hear that some of her friends are absent from her primary school due to high fever.

Dr. I see. She may have the flu. Jane, I'll do a test to see if there is any virus in your nose. You may feel a bit uncomfortable, but I want you to be brave.

Pt. Ouch!

Dr. Good girl, you are doing very well. Now, it's over. We will have the results in about 10 minutes. Please wait in the isolation room.

Dr. おはようございます．娘さんはどうされましたか．
M.（母） 急に高い熱が出て心配で連れてきました．
Dr. いつごろから，どれくらいの熱がありましたか．
M.（母） 昨日の夕方から高熱が出ました．39.4度まで上がりました．
Dr. 他に何か症状がありますか．

M.（母） 咳が出て，頭と手足が痛いといっています．おなかも痛いようですが，下痢や嘔吐はありません．とにかくしんどそうです．
Dr. わかりました．それでは診察してみましょう．ジェーン，胸を「もしもし」しますよ．シャツを上げて，胸を開けてね．背中を診るから後ろを向いてね．肺の音はきれいですね．次は耳をみますよ……中耳炎はないようです．あ

りがとう．次はお口をアーンと大きく開けてね．喉は少し赤い程度ですね．お子様の周りに似た症状の人はいますか．
M.(母) この子の小学校で高熱で休んでいる友達がいるようです．
Dr. わかりました．インフルエンザの可能性があります．ジェーン，お鼻からバイ菌がいるかどうかの検査をしますね．少し気持ちが悪いけど，頑張ってね．
Pt. 痛い！
Dr. いい子だね．よく頑張っているよ……はい検査ができましたよ．お母さん，10分位で結果が出ますから，隔離室でしばらくお待ちくださいね．

💬 Coffee Break　欧米の診療会話の特徴

1．医師の自己紹介をします(日本人医師も，状況に応じて自己紹介する場合もあります)．
　Hello, Mr.Green. I'm Dr.Sato. May I help you?

2．小児科などで，患者さんのお母さんなどへの呼びかけは，"Mom" を用いないで，名前で呼びます．「お母さん」は普通自分の母親にしか用いません．
　Mrs. Janes, your son has common cold. I'll prescribe Kampo medicine.

3．これから何をするかを知らせる表現(transitional expressions)を用います．
　Let me tell you what I am thinking.(診療の結果をお話しましょう)
　First, what I'd like you to do is 〜(まず，これからあなたにしてほしいことは〜です)
　What I'd like to do now is 〜(これからすることは〜です)

4．日本の診療でよく用いられる用語でも，さらにわかりやすい言葉(laymen's terms)で説明する傾向があります．

5．通常，外国人患者さんに対して，「〜してもよろしいでしょうか」(Is that OK with you?)という表現より，「〜します」「〜しましょう」(I'll 〜, I'd like to 〜. Let me 〜, You need〜)と断言する表現のほうが多いようです．

(例)
an echo エコー	→ an ultrasound wave picture	halitosis 口臭	→ bad breath
jaundice 黄疸	→ yellow skin	conjunctivitis 結膜炎	→ pink eye
urticaria じんましん	→ hives	aortic stenosis 大動脈狭窄	→ an abnormal narrowing of the aorta
dental caries 虫歯	→ decayed tooth		

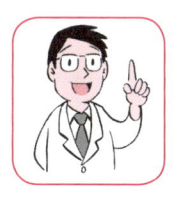

小児科

パターン7
指示

1 Please keep a fever chart (an asthma diary/a food allergy diary/ a defecation diary/a voiding diary).
熱型表（喘息日誌・食物アレルギー日誌・排便日誌・排尿日誌）をつけてください．

2 **When** you go outside, please wear a mask. **When** you get home, please wash your hands with soap and gargle thoroughly.
外出時はマスクをつけ，家に帰ったら，うがいをして，よく手を洗ってください．

3 **If** you touch vomit or loose stools, wash your hands immediately.
吐いたものや下痢便に触ったら，すぐに手を洗いましょう．

4 Please deal with the vomit using diluted hypochlorous acid or hot water.
吐いたものは，薄めた次亜塩素酸や熱湯などで処理しましょう．

*****School related ****

5 Don't go to school, **because** it's contagious.
周囲の方にうつりやすいので，学校（園など）は休みましょう．

6 He needs to take about a week off to recover.
1週間ぐらい休む必要があるでしょう．

He can**not** go back to school, **until** at least two days after the fever has gone down.　2日間以上熱が下がれば登校してもかまいません．

7 The incubation period of this disease is about two to three weeks.
潜伏期間はおよそ2〜3週間です．

During that time, your other children could get it, **so** please keep an eye on them as well.
その間，御兄弟にもうつる可能性がありますから，注意してあげてくださいね．

8 Please come again the day after tomorrow **unless** her condition changes for the worse.
状態が悪くならないようでしたら，あさって再受診してください．

If she does get worse, please bring her here immediately.
もし状態が悪くなるようなら，直ちに受診してください．

Easy talk！ 少し長い説明をする

> Step1　主語述語を確認しながら短文に切り
> Step2　主語を補いながら，
> Step3　接続詞で続けます．

日本語では，しばしば，one sentence の中で主語が異なっていても，述語がそのまま続く場合があります．

［例1］　P.61 の 5. では，「周囲の方にうつりやすい(V1)ので，学校は休ませましょう(V2)．」
　　　　　　　　　　　　　　　　　Ａ　　　　　　　Step1 ここで切って　Ｂ

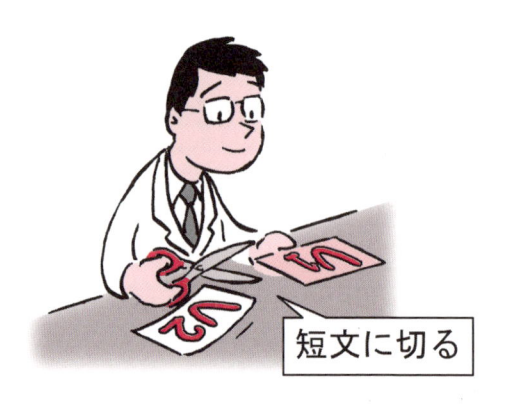

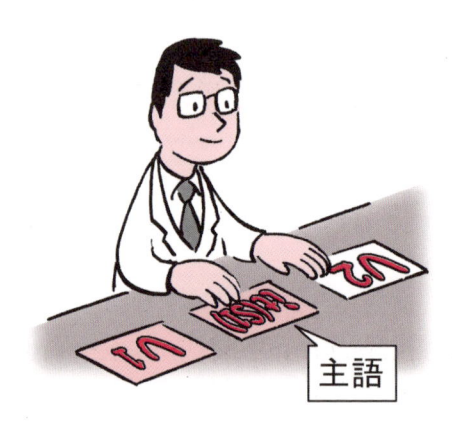

Ａ 「周囲の方に移りやすい」の Step2 主語は病気(it)ですから it(S1)を補い，
　⇒ It's contagious

Ｂ 「学校は休みましょう」は，命令文なので，⇒ don't go to school

62

Step3 接続詞（**because**）で 2 文を続け，
⇒ Don't go to school, **because** it's contagious.

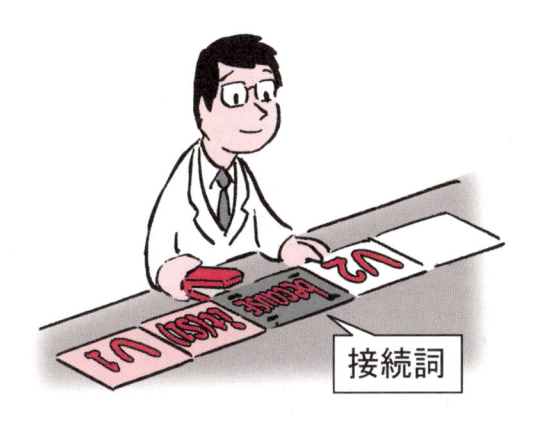

[例 2]　もう少し長い文で練習してみましょう．
「症状が(S1)治まり(V1)，状態が(S2)落ち着いていれ(V2)ば，学校に行ってもかまいません(V3)．」

　　　　　　Step1　(S)(V)を考えながら短文に切って
　　　　　　Step2　主語 She(S3)子供を補い，
　　　　　　Step3　接続詞，いれば⇒ once（いったん〜すれば）で文をつなぎ，

⇒ Once her symptoms have subsided and her condition stabilizes, she may be permitted to return to school.

■接続詞の活用：接続詞はいろいろな日本語に活用でき，日本語に引きずられないで，話す内容からどの接続詞を使えばよいかを選択します．

例 1)　When you hear the sound, please raise your right hand. 音が聞こえたら（時），右手を挙げてください．

例 2)　If he seems to be having trouble listening to the TV, please do this test. テレビの音が聞こえにくそうだったら，このテストをしてください．（もしという意味が入ります．）

例 3)　Because I have been feeling discomfort in my stomach, I had the tests. 胃にずっと不快感があり（あったので），検査しました．

例 4)　I had gastrointestinal tests and then was admitted to the hospital. 胃腸の検査をして（それから）入院しました．（単に時間的な経過を表す．）

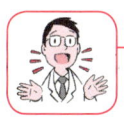

練 習　このパターンでこれだけ話せる！　　　（解答は別冊）

88.　登校可能かどうか確認しますので，1 週間後にお越しください．
89.　夜間，もしお子様の呼吸が苦しくなったらこの吸入薬を使ってください．それでも良くならなければ，急病センターを受診してください．
90.　けいれん発作が 10 〜 15 分以上続く場合や繰り返す場合は，すぐに病院へ連れてきてください．

Case 7-2　インフルエンザ（7歳女児）

Dr. Thank you for waiting. I have a positive result on the fluA test. Anti-influenza drugs are still effective if taken half a day after the development of the symptoms, so we must begin treatment promptly. May I prescribe her Tamiflu®?

M. Tamiflu®? I have heard about potential side effects through the media. Is it really safe? Are there any other effective drugs for this?

Dr. There is no evidence of a causal relationship between the drug and abnormal behavior in children. However, in view of her age (7 years old), I'd prescribe inhaled drugs like Relenza® (Zanamivir), to which fewer viruses confer resistance than to Tamiflu® and, is therefore considered effective. Maoto, Kampo medicine, is considered effective as well.

M. I don't want her to take Tamiflu®, and she can't take Kampo medicine. But I think she can use inhaled medicines. Would you please give her Relenza®?

Dr. Okay. I'll prescribe her Relenza®. Please start having her inhale it in the morning and evening soon after you get home. Although it is rare/Very occasionally, influenza can cause severe complications such as encephalopathy (a serious and potentially fatal brain disorder) and pneumonia.
Furthermore, children suffering from influenza might behave abnormally regardless of whether or not they have taken Tamiflu® or Relenza®. So please keep your eye on her. Now I'll also give her cough medicine (antitussive) and a fever reducer (antifebrile medications). However, a fever is not always a bad sign. Please do not overuse the fever reducer (antifebrile medications).

M. I understand.

Dr. Would you please call her school and inform them that she has the flu.
Please keep her home for at least two days after her fever goes down, and then once her symptoms subside and her condition stabilizes, she may return to school. Also give her enough fluids and rest. Please come again the day after tomorrow unless her condition changes for the worse. If she does

get worse, please bring her here immediately.

> **Dr.** お待たせしました．お母さん，A 型のインフルエンザ陽性の結果が出ました．発症後半日くらいなので抗インフルエンザ薬が有効だと思います．ですから，すぐに治療を始めましょう．タミフル®を処方してもよろしいでしょうか．
>
> **M.**（母）タミフル®ですか．マスコミで，タミフル®の副反応について聞いていますが，大丈夫ですか．他の薬はありませんか．
>
> **Dr.** 今のところ，子供のタミフル®服用と異常行動との因果関係を示すエビデンスはありません．7 歳ですので吸入薬のリレンザ®を処方できます．リレンザ®は，タミフル®と比較し耐性ウイルスが少なく，効果は良好とされています．それに，漢方薬の麻黄湯（まおうとう）も効果があります．
>
> **M.**（母）この子にタミフル®は使いたくないですし，漢方薬はうまく飲めません．お薬の吸入はできると思います．リレンザ®をお願いします．
>
> **Dr.** わかりました．リレンザ®を処方しますから，帰宅したらすぐに朝晩の吸入を始めてください．インフルエンザは，まれに，肺炎や脳症などの重症合併症を引き起こす場合があります．また，インフルエンザにかかっている子供は，タミフル®やリレンザ®を使わなくても異常行動を起こす場合があります．ですから，お子様から目を離さないようにしてくださいね．咳止めと解熱剤も出しておきますが，発熱は必ずしも悪いわけではありません．使い過ぎないようにしてくださいね．
>
> **M.**（母）わかりました．
>
> **Dr.** 学校には A 型インフルエンザと連絡して，休ませてください．熱が下がってから少なくとも 2 日間は家にいてください．症状が治まり，状態が落ち着いていれば学校に行ってもかまいません．お家では水分をよく摂って，安静にしてください．特に変わりがないようでしたら，あさって再受診してください．もし状態が悪くなったら早めに受診してくださいね．

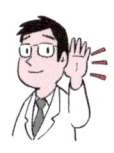

Listening comprehension （解答は別冊）

Please write true(T) or false(F).
The doctor told the patient that
91. influenza can cause encephalopathy and pneumonia. （　　）
92. children suffering influenza could behave abnormally, in association with Tamiflu or Relenza. （　　）

パターン 8

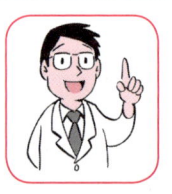

授乳についての問診

1. Does your baby 〜?　赤ちゃんは〜　しますか.
2. Do you usually 〜?　あなたはいつも〜していますか.
   Did you 〜?　あなたは〜しましたか.
3. Have you (ever) had 〜?　これまでに，あなたは〜していますか.
4. Any problems with 〜?　〜に困りますか.

例 1　Does your baby refuse breast milk or formula?　母乳かミルクを嫌がりますか.
　　　How many times a day does your baby eat weaning foods?
　　　離乳食は一日に何回あげていますか.

例 2　Have you started with weaning foods?　離乳食は始めましたか.
　　　Do you usually breastfeed or formula feed?
　　　いつもは母乳をあげますか，それともミルクですか.

例 3　How many weeks or months have you breastfed?
　　　これまで，何週間または何ヵ月母乳をあげていましたか.

例 4　Any problems with breastfeeding?　母乳をあげるのに困りますか.

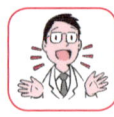

練習　このパターンでこれだけ話せる！　　　（解答は別冊）

93. ミルクはよく飲みますか.
94. 母乳は栄養面でもスキンシップとしても，とても大切です．このまま母乳を続けましょう．
95. お子様の発育と発達が良好であることを確認するために，次は10ヵ月健診にお越しください．
96. 母乳栄養でしたか，それとも人工栄養をあげましたか.
97. 離乳食は一日何回食べていますか.

あてはめましょう！

次の枠内に下記の用語をあてはめて，症状を尋ねてください．

Any problems ☐ ?
問題がありますか．（困っていますか）

with breathing 呼吸で，with infection 感染症で，with yellow skin 黄色い皮膚で（黄疸），
with labor 分娩で，having bowel movements 便通に，urinating 排尿に

Case 8-1　尿路感染症（生後 5 ヵ月男児）

Dr. Good morning. What can I do for your baby today?

M. His temperature has increased to 39 degrees and he has refused milk.

Dr. When did you first notice an increase in temperature?

M. Yesterday.

Dr. Do you breastfeed or formula feed?

M. I have used formula since he was born.

Dr. I see. Have you noticed any cold symptoms such as a cough or runny nose?

M. No, I have not. But he has vomited. I am worried because he looks lethargic and has become more cranky.

Dr. I see. Now I'll examine him. Please let me listen to his chest.
His chest sounds are clear and he has neither a red throat nor otitis media (a middle ear infection). Now could you lay him on the bed.

Dr. おはようございます．今日お子様はどうされましたか．
M.（母）39度の高熱が出て，ミルクを飲まなくなりました．
Dr. いつ頃から熱が出たのに気が付きましたか．
M.（母）昨日からです．
Dr. これまで母乳栄養ですか，人工栄養ですか．
M.（母）生まれてからずっと人工栄養でした．
Dr. わかりました．それでは，咳，鼻水などのかぜ様の症状はありましたか．
M.（母）いいえ，かぜ症状はありませんでしたが，一度嘔吐しました．元気がなく，機嫌が悪いのが心配です．
Dr. わかりました．それでは診察してみましょう．お子様の胸を診せてください．肺の音も正常で（胸部所見には異常はなく），のども赤くないですし，中耳炎もないようですね．それでは，お子様をベッドにあおむけに寝させてください．

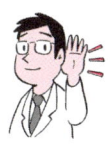

Listening comprehension　　　　　　　　（解答は別冊）

98. What is the patient's complaint? Please choose the correct ones.
   A. low-grade fever,　B. ill-temper,　C. vomiting,　D. cold symptoms

Case 8-2 尿路感染症（生後 5 ヵ月男児）

Dr. On physical examination, I don't see anything unusual. But, I am concerned about his high fever, so I want to do a blood test. May I prick his finger to run the blood test?

M. Yes, sure.

Dr. OK, then, please place his left index finger here and hold it firmly. Thank you.

〔*The Doctor pricks his finger with a tiny needle and draws blood into a capillary tube (a blood drawing instrument)*〕.

Please press this alcohol pad here for about 3 minutes to stop the bleeding. It will take about 10 minutes to get the results.

〔*10 minutes later*〕

The blood test shows an elevated WBC count of 14,700/mm^3 and C-reactive protein (CRP) levels, known as a general inflammation indicator, of 4.2mg/dl. These results show that he is most likely suffering from a bacterial infection.

Chances are that he may have a urinary tract infection. Therefore, he needs to have a urine test as well. A baby is unable to collect urine on his own, so I would like to perform a urethral catheterization to run a precise test. May I insert a fine tube (catheter) into his urethra?

M. Yes, please go ahead.

〔*The doctor examines the urine macroscopically during the catheterization.*〕

Dr. His urine appears a bit cloudy. Could you please wait until we get the results.

〔*20 minutes later*〕

His white blood cell count in urine become elevated, which indicates that he may have a urinary tract infection or UTI. Now I'll begin the treatment for a UTI. I'll need to perform a coronary count test later to confirm the UTI.

小児科

Dr. 診察上，特に異常はないようですね．熱が高いのが気になりますので，簡単な血液検査をしましょう．お子さまの指を刺して血液検査をしてもよろしいですか．

M.（母） はい．

Dr. では，左手の人指し指を出して，しっかり押さえてください．ありがとうございます．
〔細い針で指を穿刺し，キャピラリー（微量採血用の毛細管）に採血しながら〕血が止まるまで3分間くらいアルコール綿を押さえていてください．結果は10分間くらいで出ます．
〔10分後〕
血液検査では，白血球数が 14,700/mm³ と増加していて，さらに CRP という炎症反応も 4.2 mg/dl と上昇しています．この結果からすると，細菌感染症の可能性が高いようです．尿路感染症の可能性もありますから，おしっこを調べる必要があります．赤ちゃんは自分でおしっこを採ることができないので，導尿して正確なおしっこの検査をしたいと思います．お母さん，尿道に細い管を入れて検査しますが，よろしいでしょうか．

M.（母） お願いします．
〔導尿しながら，尿をみて〕

Dr. おしっこが少し濁っているようですね．尿の検査結果が出るまでしばらくお待ちください．
〔20分後〕
尿の白血球が増えていますので，尿路感染症のようですね．とりあえず，尿路感染症として治療を始めましょう．あとで今採った尿のコロニーカウントという検査をして，尿路感染症の確定診断をしましょう．

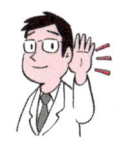

Listening comprehension　　　　　（解答は別冊）

99. Why does the doctor want to do a blood test?
100. What is the most likely diagnosis?

Case 8-3　尿路感染症（生後5ヵ月男児）

M. What are you going to do to help him?

Dr. The principal treatment is antibiotics. Considering the age of your child, I recommend that he have IV antibiotics. They may rarely cause allergic reactions. May I give him IV antibiotics?

M. Certainly, please.
〔*After starting IV*〕

Dr. Now I'll add antibiotics via a drip infusion bottle. We will monitor him, but, if you notice anything unusal such as rashes or vomiting, please let a nurse know.

M. I understand.
〔*After IV administration*〕

Dr. I think the IV will improve his condition. I'll also prescribe oral antibiotics and a fever reducers (antifebrile medication). Please bring him here tomorrow morning.

M. How do you advise me to look after him at home? (What should I do for him at home?)

Dr. Make sure he gets enough milk and water. If his condition remains poor, please bring him in again this afternoon, he may need to be hospitalized.

M. I understand. Thank you.

Dr. Please keep a good eye on him.

M.（母）　治療はどのようになりますでしょうか．

Dr.　治療は抗生物質の投与が中心になります．お子様は，年齢が小さいので，抗生剤の点滴をした方がよいと思います．抗生剤の点滴で，ごくまれにアレルギー反応がおこる場合もありますが，抗生剤の点滴をしてもよろしいでしょうか．

M.（母）　よろしくお願いします．

〔点滴開始後〕

Dr.　それでは点滴に抗生剤を入れます．こちらでもチェックしますが，もしぶつぶつが出たり，嘔吐など何か異常があれば，看護師までお知らせください．

M.（母）　わかりました．

〔点滴終了後〕

Dr.　点滴で状態が改善すると思います．抗生剤と解熱剤を処方しておきますので，．明日の朝必ず再受診してください．

M.（母）　家では何を気をつけたらよろしいですか．

Dr.　抗生剤を忘れずに飲ませて，ミルクや水分（イオン水）を十分飲ませてください．もし状態が悪いままでしたら，今日の午後もう一度受診してください．その場合は，入院が必要になるかも知れません．

M.（母）　よく分かりました．ありがとうございました．

Dr.　それでは，しっかり観察してあげてくださいね．

【翌日，尿中コロニーカウントの検査結果にて大腸菌（E.Coli）1×10^6/ml であり，急性腎盂腎炎と確定診断された．外来での抗生剤の内服と抗生剤の3日間連続点滴静注にて急性腎盂腎炎は治癒した．その後，腹部超音波検査と排尿時膀胱尿道造影検査（VCG）にて，左膀胱尿管逆流症3度と診断された．保存的治療の結果，急性腎盂腎炎の再発もなく，1年後に VUR は消失した．】

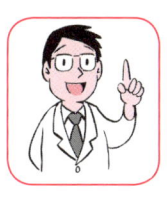

小児科

パターン9
健診時の問診

1. Can your baby 〜?/Is your baby able to 〜?　〜ができますか．
2. At what age did your baby 〜?　何歳で〜しましたか．
   When did your baby 〜?　いつ〜しましたか．

例1　Is your baby able to hold his head and neck stable?　首は据わっていますか．
例2　Is he able to sit up by himself?　自分でお座りができますか．
　　　At what age did he sit up?　何歳でお座りができましたか．
例3　Is he able to roll over both ways?　寝返りができますか．
　　　At what age did he roll over?　何歳で寝返りをしましたか．
例4　Is he able to crawl?　ハイハイはできますか．
　　　When did he start crawling?　いつハイハイを始めましたか．
例5　Can he walk by holding onto a table?　伝い歩きができますか．
例6　Can he pull himself up without assistance?　ひとり立ちができますか．
例7　Can he make sounds, such as "ba," "da," or "ma"?　「ば」「だ」「ま」などの音を発しますか．

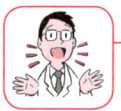

練習　このパターンでこれだけ話せる！　（解答は別冊）

101．目でおもちゃを追うことができますか．
102．音のするほうに顔を向けますか．
103．2語文が言えますか．
104．「ママ」「パパ」などの単語がいえますか．
105．おもちゃを手でつかみますか．
106．ストローで水が飲めますか．
107．友達と同じように遊びますか．
108．定期健診を受けていますか．

💬 **Coffee Break**

生後1ヵ月か2ヵ月くらいでは，ウー（"ooh"s）やアー（"ahh"s）などの音を発し（babbling），その後，ママ，ダダ（"mama" and "dada"）に変わった後，ママやパパ（"mama or dad"）といった言葉を話すことができるようになります．

Case 9-1 乳幼児健診（生後 10 ヵ月男児）

[After submitting a 10 month well-baby checkup card and Maternal and Child Health Handbook (Boshi-techo) and questionnaire, and having her baby's height and weight measured, a woman enters the consultation room with him]

Dr. Hello. Your baby is now 10 months old. Time really flies.

M. Yes, he eats baby food well.

[The doctor reviews the questionnaire]

Dr. His height and weight seems to be progressing well. His Kaup index is 17.0, which indicates that he is in the normal course of children's growth. He seems to be able to stand with support, but would you please tell me if he can walk without assistance.

M. Yes, he can. He can walk two or three steps without support.

Dr. That's fantastic! He also seems to be babbling, saying "dada and baba". I'm going to examine him. Please take his clothes off, except for his diaper. He has infantile eczema on his face and body. Are you applying any medicines to this?

M. Yes, I am applying skin care products to his skin. It has gotten much better.

Dr. OK, please continue with the ointments. The heart and lungs are clear to auscultation. Two upper and lower teeth have already grown and there is nothing unusual in his mouth.

〔受付で10ヵ月健診の問診票，母子手帳などを提出後，体重，身長，胸囲，頭囲などの計測を終えて，健診室に入っている〕

Dr. お子さんはもう10ヵ月になりましたね．本当に早いですね．

M.(母) おかげさまで，離乳食もよく食べてくれます．

〔問診票を見ながら〕

Dr. 身長も体重も順調に増えているようですね．カウプ指数も17.0とバランスも良好です．つかまり立ちはできるようですが，伝い歩きはできますか．

M.(母) はい，伝い歩きもできます．2〜3歩なら一人で歩けます．

Dr. それはすばらしいですね！「ダダ，ババ」とか発語ができるようですね．それでは診察をしてみましょう．おむつだけにして，抱っこしてください．顔と体に乳児湿疹がありますが，お薬を塗っていますか．

M.(母) はい．スキンケアをしています．前よりだいぶよくなりました．

Dr. その軟膏を続けて塗ってください．聴診では心肺には異常はありませんね．上下に歯が2本ずつ生えていて，口の中も，特に異常はないようです．

小児科

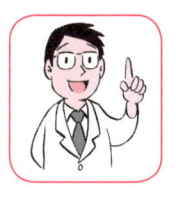

パターン 10
健診時の指示

1. From the perspectives of nutrition, immunity, and bonding, breast milk is the best. Please persevere with breastfeeding.
   栄養学的にも，免疫学的にもスキンシップの上でも，母乳が一番です．ぜひ母乳を続けましょう．

2. Please tell your husband to refrain from smoking, as passive smoke is potentially harmful to your child.
   お父さんのたばこは，お子様にも影響がありますからやめましょう．

3. Please consult a nutritionist.　栄養相談を受けてください

4. Please keep your child from having accidents and injuries, including falls, accidental ingestion, suffocation, bruises, wounds, and burns.
   転倒，異物誤飲，窒息，打撲，外傷，熱傷などの事故や外傷に気をつけましょう．

5. Please limit how much your child watches television or videos.
   テレビやビデオは控えましょう．

Case 9-2　乳幼児健診（生後 10 ヵ月男児）

Dr. Lay your son on the bed facing up. I don't see anything wrong with his abdomen. Both testes are descended. He seems to have suffered a bit from diaper dermatitis, so please apply the ointment or cream here as well.
〔*The doctor stands the baby up*〕His feet and his back are also fine.
〔*The doctor leans the baby forward*〕Both his growth and development are going very well. Do you have any concerns?

M. What I am concerned about is he is getting so active that he might get hurt.

Dr. Well, statistically, babies of around 10 months are most likely to have accidents, like falling down and hitting their head, getting burned, or drinking something harmful. The important thing is to prevent accidents. I'll give you this copy of a safety check sheet. You can check for yourself to see if he is safe. Do you let your baby watch television?

M. Yes, I do. When he is alone or eating something, I usually turn on the television.

Dr. OK. Recently, it's been shown that television may be quite harmful to babies. Please let him watch as little TV as possible. Instead, please play with or cradle him. It's also a good idea to read a picture book to him.

M. I see. I'll talk about it with my husband and try to play with him more.

Dr. Please come again for the one-year well-baby checkup when he receives his MR vaccination.

Dr. ベッドにあおむけに寝させてください．お腹に異常はありません．精巣も両方とも降りているようですね．おむつのところが，すこしかぶれているようなので，陰部もスキンケアしてください．
〔乳児を立たせるようにしながら〕足腰はしっかりしていますね．背骨にも異常はないようです．
〔乳児をゆっくりと前に倒しながら〕発育も発達も，大変順調に育っていますよ．他に，何かご心配なことはありますか．

M.（母）心配なことと言えば，よく動くようになり，けがが心配です．

Dr. そうですね．統計上も，10ヵ月ごろが一番事故が多い月齢です．落ちて頭を打ったり，やけどをしたり，誤飲したりすることがあります．事故は予防が肝心です．このコピーをお渡ししますから，安全かどうかをチェックしてみてください．それと，テレビは見せていますか．

M.（母）はい，食事の時や，一人でいる時などテレビをつけています．

Dr. そうですか．最近，テレビは赤ちゃんには害はあっても益はないことがわかってきました．テレビはできるだけ見せないようにしましょう．そのかわり，よくあやしてください．絵本を読んであげるのもよいでしょう．

M.（母）わかりました，夫とも相談してスキンシップにつとめます．

Dr. では，1歳の健診にお越しください．その時に，MRワクチンを受けてください．

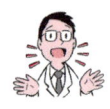

Listening comprehension　　　　　　　　　　（解答は別冊）

109. What did the doctor say of the baby's growth and development? Please choose the correct one.

　　A. not good　　B. normal　　C. very good

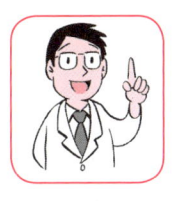

小児科

パターン 11
予防接種時の会話

1. We can do the immunization today. Please sign the consent form.
   予防接種ができますから，同意書にサインしてください．

2. I am going to administer the vaccine to your left arm.
   左の腕に予防接種をします．

3. After immunization, you should remain in the clinic for at least 30 minutes. If anything unusual occurs, please inform a nurse immediately.
   予防接種のあと，30分はクリニックにいてください．何かあれば，すぐに看護師までお知らせください．

4. Four weeks from now, we will administer the MR vaccine.
   次は，4週後にMRワクチンを受けてください．

5. Voluntary vaccinations, including the mumps and varicella vaccines, are likewise recommended.
   おたふくかぜ，水痘ワクチンなどの任意予防接種はできればお受けください．

words & expressions

Maternal Child Health book 母子手帳　vaccination coupons and questionnaire 予防接種券と予診票
regular vaccinations 定期接種
diphtheria-pertussis-tetanus combined 三種混合(DPT)ジフテリア・百日咳・破傷風
diphtheria-tetanus combined 二種混合(DT)
measles-rubella combined 麻疹・風疹(MR)
Japanese encephalitis 日本脳炎
voluntary vaccinations 任意接種
mumps おたふくかぜ　varicella 水痘　Hib ヒブ
streptococcus pneumonia 肺炎連鎖球菌
influenza インフルエンザ
cervical cancer 子宮頚がん
hepatitis B (HB) B型肝炎

Case 10-1   流行性耳下腺炎（5歳男児）

Dr. Hello. What can I do for you today?

M. His right cheek has been swollen and painful since yesterday. He seems to have a slight cough as well.

Dr. His right cheek (parotid gland) looks greatly swollen. He also has a slight fever of 37.8. Please let me examine him.

〔*After auscultation.*〕 His lungs seem clear. Now, please open your mouth wide.

〔*The child winces in pain upon opening his mouth.*〕

M. He said that his mouth has been hurting a bit when he eats. This has been going on since yesterday.

〔*The doctor palpates the right parotid area.*〕

Dr. Now, I am going to push here slowly, so please tell me when it hurts.

〔*The child recoils in pain.*〕

Dr. Then, how about here?

〔*The child again recoils from the pain.*〕

Dr. Ok. He seems to have parotitis. Does anyone else around him have similar symptoms?

M. Yes, I heard that a few children are suffering from mumps in his class.

Dr. For how long?

M. For about one to two weeks. Several of his friends seem to have it as well.

Dr. こんにちは．どうされましたか．

M.（母） 昨日から，右の頬が腫れてきました．痛みもあるようです．少し咳も見られます．

Dr. 右の耳下腺部分がだいぶ腫れていますね．熱は37.8度とやや高めですね．それでは診察してみましょう．〔聴診後〕胸には，特に異常はないようです．お口を大きく開けてくださいね．
〔患児は口をあけながら痛みを訴える〕

M.（母） 昨日からずっと，ご飯を食べる時口が痛いと言っていました．

〔右の耳下腺部分を触れながら〕

Dr. 今度は，ここをゆっくり押さえてみるからね．痛かったら教えてね．
〔患児は，痛いと反応した〕

Dr. ここはどうですか．
〔患児は再び痛がった〕

Dr. いいですよ．おかあさん，耳下腺炎のようです．まわりに，どなたか，同じような症状の方がいらっしゃいませんでしたか．

M.（母） はい，この子の幼稚園ではおたふくかぜの子がいると聞いていますが・・・

Dr. それは，どれくらい前からですか．
M.（母） 1〜2週間だと思います．何人かのお友達が，おたふくかぜにかかったようです．

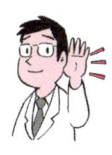

Listening comprehension
（解答は別冊）

110. What are the patient's complaints? Please choose the correct ones.
    A. high fever
    B. pain
    C. persistent cough
    D. swelling in the left cheek

Case 10-2　流行性耳下腺炎（5歳男児）

Dr. I see. Did your son get immuninized with the mumps vaccine?

M. No, he didn't get it. He's never had mumps.

Dr. I see. Taking his circumstances into consideration, he may well have epidemic parotitis, or as it is commonly called mumps. Here, recurrent parotitis (an inflammation of the parotid salivary glands) cannot be ruled out, because he mainly complains of swelling over the right parotid area.

M. What is recurrent parotitis?

〔The doctor shows an instructional leaflet to the patient〕

Dr. As shown here, both diseases are conditions that cause swelling over the parotid glands. Mumps refers to epidemic parotitis caused by the mumps virus.

M. Can you tell me which one he has?

Dr. At this stage, I can't tell you which one he has with 100% certainty. If we do an ultrasound test, it may help distinguish between the two diagnoses.

M. I see. Would it be possible to do the test today? It's more convenient for us, given my work and kindergarten schedules.

Dr. Ok, I will prepare for it.

Dr. お子様は，おたふくかぜワクチン接種はされていますか．

M.（母） おたふくかぜのワクチンはしていません．おたふくかぜにかかったこともありません．

Dr. そうですか．まわりの状況も考えると流行性耳下腺炎つまりおたふくかぜの可能性が高いようです．今のところ，右の耳下腺の腫れが主なようなので，反復性耳下腺炎の可能性も否定しきれません．

M.（母） 反復性耳下腺炎とはどのような病気ですか．

〔医師は説明書を見せながら〕

Dr. このように，どちらも耳下腺が腫れる病気で

す．おたふくかぜウイルスによる耳下腺炎のみがおたふくかぜといわれています．
M.（母）　どちらかわかりませんか．
Dr.　今の段階で完全に鑑別することはできませんが，超音波検査をすれば，どちらの病気か，ある程度の鑑別ができると思います．
M.（母）　そうですか．子供の幼稚園や仕事の都合がありますので，今日，検査していただけますか．
Dr.　わかりました．それでは，これから準備しましょう．

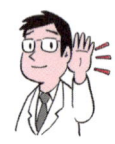

Listening comprehension

（解答は別冊）

111. Why does the doctor say the patient may have mumps, or recurrent parotitis?

Case 10-3　流行性耳下腺炎（5歳男児）

〔*During the ultrasound examination*〕

M. How do things look?

Dr. The results show that he may have mumps. Please inform his kindergarten of the diagnosis and keep him home for a while.

M. I see. How long should he be kept away from kindergarden?

Dr. It depends on his condition, but he cannot go back to his kindergarten until the swelling goes away. It may take 7 days or so.

M. Does it take that long? Is there anything else I should be careful about?

Dr. It's known that mumps may cause complications, including meningitis, pancreatitis, and orchitis. Please watch him carefully and check to see if headaches, stomach aches, or testicular pain develop. Mumps can also very occasionally cause hearing disturbances. There is a test to find out about hearing difficulties at an early stage. This test can be done at your home. I'll show you how to do it.

〔*After confirmation of his hearing ability in both ears*〕

Dr. His hearing seems to be fine and intact. If you notice that he begins to have trouble listening to the TV or conversation, please try this test. There is no medicine that is directly effective for the mumps virus, so I am going to give him some cough medicine and antifebrile. If you don't notice any change in his condition, please return in 3 days so we can re-evaluate his condition.

〔*超音波検査をしながら*〕
M.（母）　どうでしょうか．
Dr.　検査結果からは，おたふくかぜの可能性が高いようです．幼稚園には，おたふくかぜと連絡して，しばらく休ませてください．
M.（母）　わかりました．どれくらい休む必要がありますか．
Dr.　症状にもよりますが，耳下腺の腫れが引くまで園には行かれません．7日前後かかるかも知れません．
M.（母）　そんなにかかりますか．他に気をつけることはありませんでしょうか．
Dr.　おたふくかぜは，髄膜炎や膵炎，精巣炎などの合併症があります．頭痛，腹痛，精巣痛などに注意してください．また，稀に，難聴をきたすことがあります．難聴を早く見つけられる方法があります．お家でもできますよ．テストのやり方をお見せしましょう．
〔*患児の両側の聴力を確認後*〕
お母さん，今は非常によく聞こえているようです．テレビの音が聞こえにくかったり，会話が聞き取りにくいようでしたら，このテストをしてみてください．直接おたふくかぜに効くお薬はないので，咳止めのお薬と解熱剤を出しておきます．それでは，変わりがないようでしたら，次は3日後にお越しください．その時また，検討しましょう．

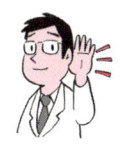

Listening comprehension

（解答は別冊）

112.　What is the most likely diagnosis?

PART 1 産婦人科

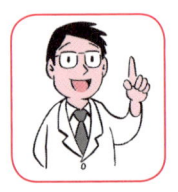

パターン1
症状について尋ねる

Do you have 症 状 ?

例　Do you have any cramps or discomfort in your lower abdomen during your period?
　　生理時に，下腹部に痛み（けいれん痛）や不快感がありますか．

Easy Talk!

基本的な英会話の骨格は内科の解説と同様に**症状**（Do you have any cramps or discomfort）のあとに症状が起こった**部位**（in your lower abdomen）最後に，**いつ**（during your period）を追加していきます．

あてはめましょう！

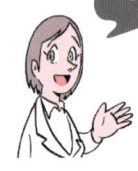

次の枠内に用語をあてはめて，症状を尋ねてください．

Do you have ☐ ?

（痛み）　any strong pain during your periods 生理時に強い痛み，any cramps in the lower abdomen 下腹痛，any pain during intercourse 性交痛，any pain in your breast 乳房痛，any lower back pain 腰痛，any genital pain 外陰痛

（その他の症状）　any itching かゆみ，any vaginal discomfort 陰部の不快感，any vaginal dryness 陰部の乾燥感，any abdominal bloating 腹部膨満感，lumps/bumps しこり，dimples 陥没

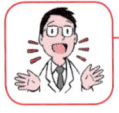

練習　このパターンでこれだけ話せる！　　（解答は別冊）

113. これまでにお腹の腫れに気がついたことはありますか．
114. 排尿時か，排便時に不快感はありますか．

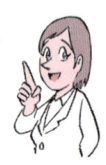

使えるパターンを増やそう！

痛みについてのその他の質問例

Where is the pain located?　どこが痛みますか．
What does the pain feel like? Stabbing, or dull?
どのような痛みですか．刺すような痛みですか，それとも鈍い痛みですか．

産婦人科

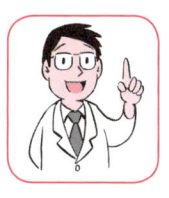

パターン2 月経／出血についての問診

1 ～しますか．

Do you have a period every month? Are your periods regular?
毎月生理はありますか．規則正しいですか．

2 いつですか．

When + was your last (menstrual) period? Was it normal?
最終月経はいつでしたか．正常でしたか．

3 どれくらい～ですか．

How many days + **did your period last**?
月経はどれくらい続きましたか．

+ **do they** (your menstrual periods) **last**?
通常の月経はどれくらい続きますか．

How long + is your typical menstrual cycle?
月経周期はどれくらいですか．

How many pads or tampons + **do you use a day**?
一日にどれくらいナプキンやタンポンを使いますか．

How heavy + is your menstrual flow? Heavy or light?
経血量はどれくらいですか．多いですかそれとも少ないですか．

4 ～したのは，何歳の時でしたか．

How old were you + **when your periods started**?
初経年齢は何歳でしたか．

+ when you had your last period?
閉経年齢は何歳でしたか．

あてはめましょう！

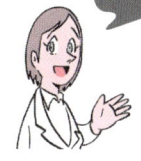

次の枠内に下記の用語をあてはめて，症状を尋ねてください．
(a) When was ☐ ?
(b) (Are there) Any ☐ ?

(a) your second to last period (from when to when)? (最終月経の)前の月経はいつですか．(いつからいつ

83

まで),
 the first day of your last period（LMP） 最終月経はいつから始まりましたか.
 your last visit to the gynecologist 婦人科の診察を最後に受けたのはいつでしたか.
(b) changes in your period recently 最近，生理に何か変わったことはありますか.
 mood swings or irritability around your period 生理ごろになると気分が動揺したり，いらいらしたりしますか.
 concerns about sexual function 性機能について心配ごとはありますか.

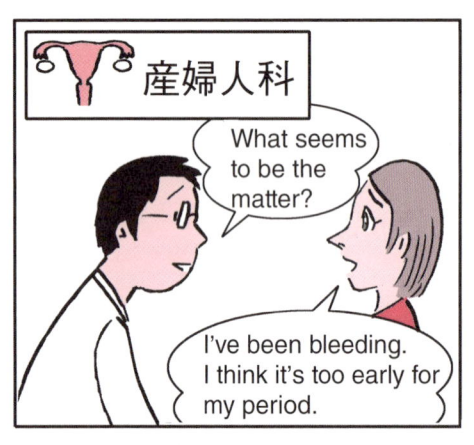

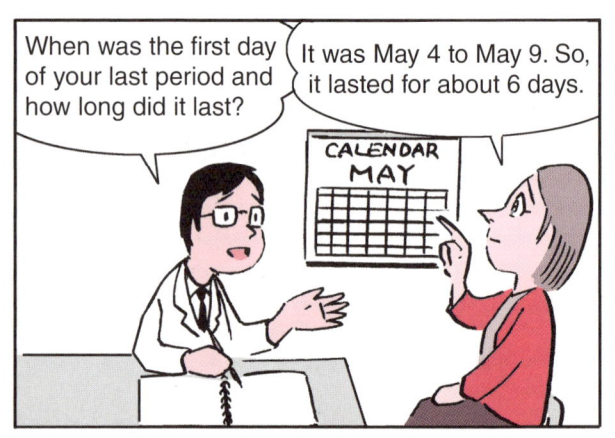

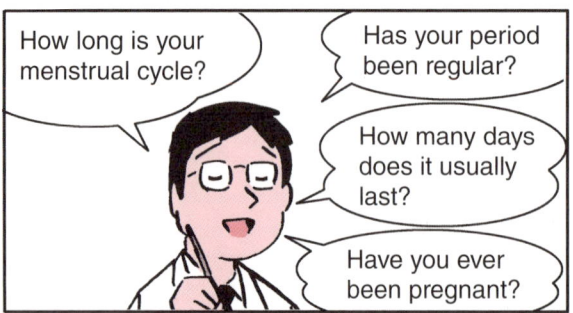

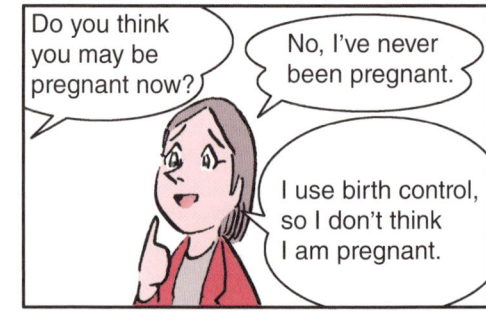

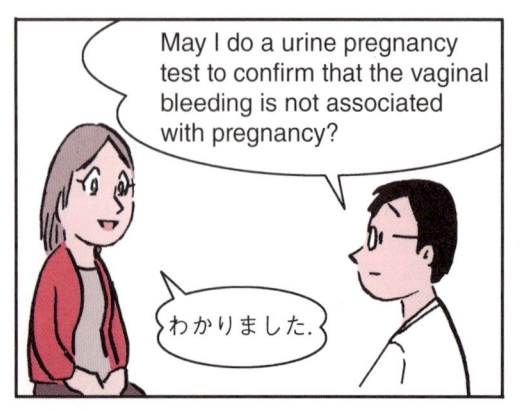

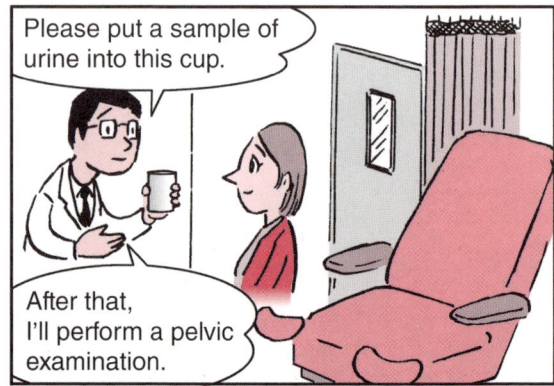

産婦人科

What seems to be the matter?

I've been bleeding. I think it's too early for my period.

When was the first day of your last period and how long did it last?

It was May 4 to May 9. So, it lasted for about 6 days.

How long is your menstrual cycle?

Has your period been regular?

How many days does it usually last?

Have you ever been pregnant?

Do you think you may be pregnant now?

No, I've never been pregnant.

I use birth control, so I don't think I am pregnant.

May I do a urine pregnancy test to confirm that the vaginal bleeding is not associated with pregnancy?

わかりました.

Please put a sample of urine into this cup.

After that, I'll perform a pelvic examination.

Case 11-1　不正出血（26歳女性）

Dr. Hello. What seems to be the matter?

Pt. I've been bleeding for the last two days. I think it is too early for my period.

Dr. Have you ever had bleeding like this before?

Pt. I've had it about once a year, outside of my usual periods.

Dr. Do you have any pain in your abdomen or genital area?

Pt. No, I don't.

Dr. When was the first day of your last period and how long did it last?

Pt. It was from May 4 to May 9. So, it lasted for 6 days.

Dr. How long is your menstrual cycle? Are they regular?

Pt. It is usually 28 to 30 days, and fairly regular.

Dr. How many days does it usually last?

Pt. It lasts for 5 or 6 days.

Dr. Are you taking any medicines at the moment, such as hormonal drugs?

Pt. No, I'm not.

Dr. Are you married?

Pt. No, I'm not.

Dr. Have you ever had sex?

Pt. Yes, I have.

Dr. Do you think this bleeding was associated with sex? For example, did you bleed after intercourse?

Pt. No, I don't think so.

Dr. Have you ever been pregnant or do you think you may be pregnant now?

Pt. No, I've never been pregnant. I use birth control, so I don't think I am pregnant.

Dr. What do you use to avoid pregnancy?

Pt. I used to take the pill, but now I always use a condom.

Dr. May I do a urine pregnancy test to confirm that the vaginal bleeding is not associated with pregnancy? Even with the use of a condom, pregnancy

may very occasionally result.
Pt. OK.
Dr. Please put a sample of urine into this cup. After that, I'll perform a pelvic examination.
Pt. I see.

Dr. こんにちは，どうされましたか．
Pt. 2日前から出血があります．まだ次の生理には早いと思うのですが．
Dr. このような出血は，はじめてですか．
Pt. 今まで1年に1回くらい，生理と違う時に出血することがありました．
Dr. お腹や陰部の痛みはないですか．
Pt. ありません．
Dr. 最後の月経は，いつからはじまって何日くらい続きましたか．
Pt. 5月4日から9日までです．ですから，6日間位続きました．
Dr. いつも月経は何日くらいの周期で来ますか．周期は規則正しいですか．
Pt. 28〜30日くらいの間隔で，大体，規則的です．
Dr. 月経出血はいつも何日くらい続きますか．
Pt. 5〜6日です．
Dr. 今，何か飲んでいるお薬はないですか．たとえば，ホルモン剤とか．
Pt. いいえ．
Dr. ご結婚されていますか．
Pt. いいえ．独身です．
Dr. セックスの経験はありますか．
Pt. はい．
Dr. 今回の出血はセックスと関係はありませんか．セックスの後に出血したとか．
Pt. いいえ．
Dr. 今まで妊娠したことはありますか．現在，妊娠している可能性はありますか．
Pt. 妊娠したことはありません．避妊しているので，今妊娠している可能性もないと思います．
Dr. どのような方法で避妊をされていますか．
Pt. 以前はピルをのんでいましたが，今はコンドームです．
Dr. 念のため，不正出血が妊娠に伴うものでないかを確認するために尿の妊娠反応をチェックさせていただいてよろしいですか．コンドームを使っていても稀に妊娠することがありますので．
Pt. わかりました．
Dr. では，コップに尿をとってください．その後，診察(内診)をさせていただきますね．
Pt. はい．

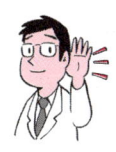

Listening comprehension (解答は別冊)

115. What kind of examination is she going to have to confirm pregnancy?

case 11-2　不正出血（26歳女性）

Dr. Please remove your underwear, change into slippers, and hop on this table right here. I'll examine you now. Please relax your abdomen. Also, please let me know if you feel discomfort or pain during the examination. OK, I'm finished. You might bleed slightly today as a result of this examination, but this is normal.

〔After the examination〕

Dr. I didn't find any diseases such as vaginitis or abnormal growths such as polyps or uterine fibroids, that could cause irregular bleeding on either the ultrasound or the internal examination. In addition, the pregnancy test is negative. I performed a Pap smear (test) to double check for uterine cancer, just in case. I think the bleeding is functional uterine bleeding, which is irregular bleeding as a result of unbalanced hormones.

Pt. What causes it?

Dr. There are various causes. Physical and mental stress can often cause your hormones to become temporarily unbalanced.

Pt. Well, recently I have not been sleeping well and my lifestyle has been very irregular, so that makes sense to me.

Dr. You may also bleed for several days due to the hormonal changes which take place during ovulation in the middle of your cycle. This is called ovulation bleeding, and you don't need to worry about it.

Pt. So, at the moment, it doesn't look like anything serious?

Dr. At this moment, no. If your irregular bleeding or irregular menstruation continues, you may need a Basal Body Temperature Measurement (BBT) and a hormone blood test. But today, the amount of bleeding is small, so let's see how things go. If you're still bleeding in a week, then it would probably be better for you to take hormones to stop it.

Pt. I see. When should I come back?

Dr. I'll discuss the results of your uterine cancer test in a week. If you have a lot of bleeding or abdominal pain before then, please come to see me as soon as possible.

Dr. 下着を外してスリッパに履き替えて，内診台に乗ってください．では診察します．お腹の力を抜いてリラックスして楽にしてください．診察中，気分が悪くなったり，痛みがあれば教えてください．これで，診察は終わりです．診察の影響で今日は少し出血が増えるかもしれませんが，心配ありません．

〔診察後〕

Dr. 内診と超音波では，腟炎やポリープ，筋腫といった不正出血の原因となるような疾患はみられませんでした．妊娠反応も陰性です．念のため子宮癌のスメア検査をしました．今回の出血はおそらく機能性出血だと思われます．機能性出血とは，ホルモンのアンバランスによる不正出血のことです．

Pt. その原因は何ですか．

Dr. 様々なものがありますが，一時的なホルモンのアンバランスは，肉体的・精神的ストレスが誘引になっていることが多いものです．

Pt. 最近，睡眠不足が続いていました．生活も不規則になっていましたので，心当たりはあります．

Dr. 月経周期のちょうど真ん中頃，排卵が起こる頃に生じるホルモンの変化のため，数日出血が起こることもあります．これは排卵期出血といって，心配のないものです．

Pt. じゃあ，さしあたって，大きな病気はなさそうですか．

Dr. はい，そう思います．これからも，不正出血や月経不順が続くようなら基礎体温測定や血中ホルモン検査も必要かもしれません．でも，今日は出血量も少ないので経過をみましょう．1週間様子を見て，出血が止まる気配がないようなら，ホルモン剤を飲んで止血した方がよいかもしれませんね．

Pt. わかりました．次はいつ受診すればいいですか．

Dr. 子宮癌の検査の結果は，1週間後に説明させていただきます．もしそれまでに大量の出血や腹痛などがあれば，早めに受診してください．

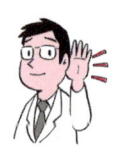

Listening comprehension

（解答は別冊）

116. What is the most likely diagnosis?

産婦人科

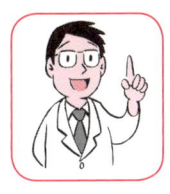

パターン3 妊娠歴／避妊についての問診

1 妊娠歴について尋ねる

Have you (ever) had an abortion or miscarriage?
中絶や流産をしたことはありますか．

Have you ever been pregnant?
妊娠したことはありますか．

Would you please tell me more about your pregnancies?
妊娠歴についてくわしく教えていただけますか．

2 妊娠回数について尋ねる

How many times ＋ have you been pregnant?
いままで何度妊娠されましたか．

3 妊娠の可能性について尋ねる

Is there any possibility of your being pregnant (right) now?

Is there any possibility that you are pregnant now?
今，妊娠している可能性はないですか．

4 避妊について尋ねる

What do you use to avoid pregnancy?
どのような方法で避妊をされていますか．

Are you currently using hormonal birth control?
今，ホルモン避妊薬を使用していますか．

あてはめましょう！

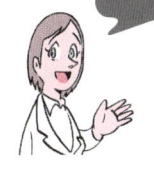

次の枠内に下記の用語をあてはめて，「(これまでに)〜したことはありますか」と尋ねてください．

Have you (ever) [　　　] ?

had an abortion or miscarriage 中絶又は流産をした．
taken a home pregnancy test 家で妊娠テストをした．
missed taking any birth control pills 避妊薬を飲み忘れた．
been under increased physical or emotional stress 肉体的精神的にストレスが増えた．
lost or gained weight 体重が増えたり減ったりした．　passed any blood clots 血塊があった．

Case 12-1　卵巣嚢腫(34歳女性)

Dr. How do you do? What seems to be the problem?

Pt. I've had a pain in my lower right abdomen for 5 days. I went to see a doctor this morning, but she said that it's not an internal organ disorder and advised me to see a gynecologist.

Dr. What sort of pain is it?

Pt. Well, at first it was stabbing. It then became a dull ache for the last 2 to 3 days.

Dr. Do you have any pain or discomfort during or after urination?

Pt. No, I don't.

Dr. Have you ever had this kind of pain before?

Pt. I've had occasional discomfort in my lower right abdomen for about 2 to 3 years.

Dr. When was your last period?

Pt. It started last Thursday, and lasted a week.

Dr. Is there any possibility of your being pregnant right now?

Pt. Well, my period just finished, but is there any chance of being pregnant?

Dr. There is still a chance. Even if you think it is menstrual bleeding, you can get vaginal bleeding during early pregnancy.

Pt. I see. But I am still sure I am not pregnant because I haven't had intercourse with my husband in a while.

Dr. はじめまして．どうされましたか．
Pt. 5日前から，右の下腹が痛いのです．今朝，内科で診察を受けたのですが，内科の病気ではないといわれ，婦人科を受診するように勧められました．
Dr. 痛みはどんな感じですか．
Pt. えーっと，はじめ，キリキリした痛みでしたが，2, 3日前からはジワジワした鈍い痛みですね．
Dr. 尿をする時や尿をした後の痛みや不快感はないですか．
Pt. ありません．
Dr. 今までこうしたことはありましたか．
Pt. 2〜3年前から時々，右の下腹が気持ち悪い時がありました．
Dr. 最後の月経はいつごろでしたか．
Pt. 先週の木曜から，1週間ありました．
Dr. 今，妊娠している可能性はないですか．
Pt. 生理が終わったところなのに，妊娠していることがあるのですか．
Dr. そうですね．月経出血と思っていたものが，妊娠初期の出血という可能性もありますから

Pt.	そうですか．でもいずれにしても妊娠の可能性はありません．しばらく夫と交渉はありませんから．

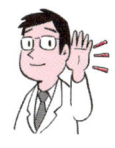

Listening comprehension

(解答は別冊)

117. What is the patient's chief complaint?

Case 12-2　卵巣囊腫（34歳女性）

- Dr. I see. Do you have strong period pains/menstrual cramps?
- Pt. I sometimes take painkillers on the second day of my periods, but not every time.
- Dr. Is your usual flow light or heavy?
- Pt. I don't know if my flow is heavier than others, but sometimes there are clots in the blood.
- Dr. When was your last visit to a gynecologist?
- Pt. It was two years ago.
- Dr. What was that visit for?
- Pt. I had a heavy vaginal discharge, so I went to see a doctor. I was diagnosed with candidiasis, and was treated with vaginal suppositories. At that time, the doctor told me that my uterus was a bit big.
- Dr. How many times have you been pregnant, and how many times have you given birth?
- Pt. I have been pregnant 4 times and given birth twice.
- Dr. Did the other two pregnancies end in abortion or miscarriage? Please tell me about your pregnancies.
- Pt. The first time I got pregnant, I was 19 years old and had an abortion. When I was 23 years old, I had miscarriage. With my third pregnancy, I had my older daughter when I was 26. And I had my second child when I was 28.
- Dr. Were your two deliveries normal? Are your children healthy?

Pt. My first delivery was normal, but it was a difficult delivery (dystocia) and the doctor used forceps. I had the second baby by Cesarean section due to placenta previa. They are both healthy.

Dr. わかりました．生理痛は強い方ですか．
Pt. 生理の 2 日目頃，生理痛の薬を飲むことがありますが，毎回ではありません．
Dr. 経血の量はいかがですか．特に多いとか，少ないとか．
Pt. 人と比べて多いのかどうかはわかりませんが，塊のような出血が出ることもあります．
Dr. 婦人科の診察を最後に受けたのはいつですか．
Pt. 2 年前です．
Dr. その時は何で受診されましたか．
Pt. おりものが多かったので診察を受けました．カンジダといわれて腟坐薬で治療しました．その時，内診で少し子宮が大きいといわれました．

Dr. いままで何度妊娠して何度出産されましたか．
Pt. 妊娠は 4 回，出産は 2 回です．
Dr. 後の 2 回は中絶ですか，流産ですか．妊娠歴をくわしく教えていただけますか．
Pt. はじめの妊娠は 19 歳の時で中絶しました．2 度目は 23 歳の時で流産．3 度目の妊娠は 26 歳でこの時に長女を出産しました．2 度目の出産は 28 歳の時です．
Dr. お産は 2 回とも正常分娩でしたか．お子様はお元気ですか．
Pt. 1 回目は正常なお産でしたが，難産で吸引分娩しました．2 回目は前置胎盤で帝王切開です．子供は二人とも健康です．

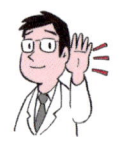

Listening comprehension (解答は別冊)

118. What was the patient told when she went to see a gynecologist due to a heavy vaginal discharge? Choose the correct one.
 A. dystocia　　B. candidiasis　　C. placenta previa

Coffee break

「女を見たら妊娠と思え」という言葉は臨床の鉄則です．女性が出血や下腹痛を訴えて受診した時には，「現在，妊娠している可能性はないですか．Is there any possibility of your being pregnant?」を忘れないようにしましょう．また妊娠中の女性に有害な検査や投薬をしないためにもこの質問は重要です．

本人が「妊娠している可能性はありません．There is no possibility of being pregnant.」と訴えた時でも，その理由が「生理が終わったところだから Because I've just finished my period.」「今，生理中だから Because I am now having my period.」「避妊をしているから Because I am using birth control.」というものであれば，あてにはなりません．本人が月経出血 (bleeding) だと思っていても実際は流産 (miscarriage) や子宮外妊娠 (ectopic pregnancy) の出血であることはしばしばです．

産婦人科

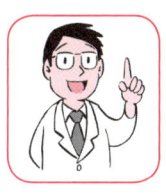

パターン4 診察時の会話

1 Please undress for the examination.
検査をしますから，衣服を脱いでください．

2 Please relax the muscles of your abdomen.　お腹の力を抜いてください．

3 Please let me know ＋ **if** you feel any pain ＋ **during** the examination.
検査の間，痛みがあれば知らせてください（→英語的語順は，知らせてください．痛みがあれば，検査の間に）（「いつ」は最後となります）．

4 I'll perform an endovaginal ultrasonography ＋ to see if the fallopian tubes are swollen.
卵管が腫れていないかを調べるために経腟超音波検査をしましょう．
I'll の代わりに，I am going to ～/let me ～など用います．

あてはめましょう！

次の枠内に下記の用語をあてはめましょう．

I'm going to/I'll ☐

inspect the vagina and cervix with a speculum. 腟鏡で内診をします（腟と頚部をみます）．
reach your cervix. 頚部に入ります．
examine some of your internal organs with my other hand. 片手で，内臓を調べます．
palpate the abdomen with my free hand. あいている手で，お腹を触診します．

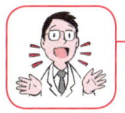

練習　このパターンでこれだけ話せる！　（解答は別冊）

119. 悪性疾患の有無を確認するために CT スキャンをしましょう．
120. 検査の間，不快感があれば，知らせてください．

Case 12-3 卵巣嚢腫(34歳女性)

Dr. I see. Now I'm going to examine your abdomen. Please lie down on this table. I'm going to press on your abdomen, so please let me know if you feel any pain.

Pt. Oh! It hurts there.

Dr. Does it hurt more when I press your abdomen or when I remove my hand?

Pt. It hurts more when you press.

Dr. Now I'm going to perform an ultrasound test, so I'll put some jelly on your abdomen. Well, your right ovary is very swollen. You have an ovarian cyst and a benign growth (uterus myoma) in your uterus. The uterine mass is rather small, so, you don't need to worry about it. I'll do an ultrasound exam through your vagina on the examination table. Let's also do a bacteriological test on your vaginal discharge to see whether there are any bacteria that can cause pelvic inflammatory disease.

Pt. What's causing the pain?

Dr. The right ovarian cyst, it seems. Just in case, I'll do tumor marker tests to rule out ovarian cancer, so please go to the laboratory to give blood samples afterward.

Pt. What is an ovarian cyst?

Dr. An ovarian cyst is a type of benign tumor with a build-up of fluid inside it.

Pt. Do I need surgery?

Dr. The size of the ovary changes depending on hormonal imbalances or the menstrual cycle. Ovarian cysts sometimes resolve on their own while we are monitoring them.

But in your case, the tumor is 8 cm across, which is big. The ultrasound findings indicate that you'll need surgery. When a swollen ovary is twisted (torsion) you may feel sudden severe abdominal pain. In that case, you may need emergency surgery. Your pain seems to be going away now, but I'll perform pre-surgery tests today.

I also recommend that you have an MRI to investigate the contents of the

産婦人科

cyst.

Pt. What kind of test is an MRI?

Dr. Magnetic resonance imaging (MRI) is a test that provides tomographic images of the body using a magnetic field and radio waves. Please make an appointment at the examination room before going home, and ask about the details of the test there.

Pt. I understand.

Dr. I'll explain the results of today's tests here in two weeks. I'll prescribe painkillers, but if you have any severe pain, please don't hesitate to phone this hospital.

Dr. わかりました．では，腹部の触診をしますので，この台に横になってください．お腹を押さえますので，痛みがあればおしえてくださいね．

Pt. あ，そこが痛いです．

Dr. 手で押さえた時と，こうして手を離した時と，どちらが痛いですか．

Pt. 押さえた時です．

Dr. では，超音波検査をします．お腹にゼリーをつけますね．
うーん，右の卵巣がかなり腫れていますね．卵巣腫瘍です．子宮筋腫もありますが，これは小さなものだから心配ないでしょう．内診台で経腟超音波検査をします．骨盤内の炎症をおこす細菌がいないかを調べるために，腟分泌物の細菌学的検査もしましょう．

Pt. 痛みの原因はなんでしょうか．

Dr. 痛みの原因は右の卵巣嚢腫だと思われます．卵巣癌の可能性も否定できないため，念のため腫瘍マーカー検査をしますので，後ほど検査室で採血を受けてください．

Pt. 卵巣嚢腫って何ですか．

Dr. 卵巣嚢腫とは，腫瘍内部に液体を溜めた良性の卵巣腫瘍です．

Pt. 手術しないといけませんか．

Dr. 卵巣は月経周期やホルモンバランスによって大きさが変化する臓器です．卵巣嚢腫も経過をみているうちに自然にしぼんで治ることがあります．あなたの嚢腫は直径が8センチと大きく，超音波所見から見ても手術が必要になる可能性が高いと思います．また，茎捻転といって，腫れた卵巣が捻れた時には突然激しい腹痛を起こすことがあります．その場合は緊急手術が必要になります．現在痛みは治まってきているようですが，手術に備え術前検査もしておきましょう．また嚢腫の性状をくわしく調べるために，MRI検査をお勧めします．

Pt. MRIとはどんな検査ですか．

Dr. 磁場と電波を用いて体の断層写真を撮る検査です．本日検査室で予約を取ってお帰りください．検査の詳細についてはそちらでお尋ねください．

Pt. わかりました．

Dr. 本日の検査結果は2週間後，外来で説明いたします．本日は鎮痛剤を処方しておきますが，激しい腹痛が起こった時には病院にお電話ください．

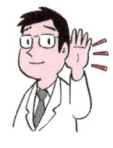

Listening comprehension （解答は別冊）

121. What is the most likely diagnosis?
122. What is the next step?

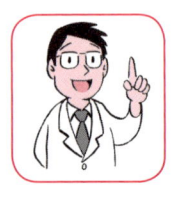

パターン5 帯下についての問診

におい
Does the vaginal discharge smell?　帯下のにおいはいかがですか．
Is there an odor associated with the discharge?　帯下にいやなにおいはありますか．

量
How much discharge do you notice? Is it heavy or light?
帯下の量はどれくらいですか．多いですか少ないですか．

色
What color is it?　帯下はどのような色ですか．

あてはめましょう！

次の枠内に下記の用語をあてはめて，症状を尋ねてください．

Is the vaginal discharge 　　　　 ?

thin さらさらしている，clear 透明な，clumpy 固まっている，blood-tinged 血が混じっている，thick like pus 膿性，frothy あわのよう，stringy 糸を引くよう，white and clumpy 白くてかたまっている，like cottage cheese カッテージチーズのよう

---

words & expressions　帯下の色の表現例

白っぽい whitish，赤褐色 dark red，褐色 dark brown，乳白色 milky，赤みがかった reddish，緑がかった greenish，茶色がかった brownish，灰色がかった grayish，黄色をおびた yellowish

Case 13　腟　炎(41歳女性)

Dr. Hello, what is troubling you?
Pt. I've been having a lot of (vaginal) discharge.
Dr. Since when?
Pt. Since about 2 to 3 months ago.
Dr. What is it like? What is its odor and color?
Pt. It's yellow and sticky, and smells a bit bad.
Dr. Is it painful or itchy?
Pt. I sometimes feel itchy. I think I may have dermatitis from the discharge.
Dr. Have you ever had similar symptoms?
Pt. No. This is the first time.
Dr. You may have a vaginal infection. I'm going to examine you to check your discharge. Please get on the table. Now I'll give you an internal examination. I'll insert a speculum, so please relax your abdomen. Next, I am going to perform tests for bacteria and a cell test for uterine cancer. That's it for the examination. Finally, I'll clean out your vagina and insert a vaginal suppository. Your discharge may increase as the suppository dissolves later, but that's nothing to worry about.

Dr. こんにちは，いかがされました．
Pt. おりものが多いのです．
Dr. いつごろからですか．
Pt. 2, 3ヵ月前からです．
Dr. どんな感じのおりものですか．色や匂いはいかがですか．
Pt. 黄色くてネバネバして，ちょっと臭いです．
Dr. 痛みや痒みはありませんか．
Pt. 時々痒いです．おりものからかぶれたのかもしれませんが．
Dr. 以前，同じような症状があったことはありますか．
Pt. いいえ，はじめてです．
Dr. 腟炎が考えられますね．内診をして，おりものを調べてみましょう．台の上にあがってください．では内診します．腟鏡を入れますのでお腹の力を抜いてください．細菌の検査と子宮癌の細胞診をします．これで検査は終わりです．腟洗浄して中に腟坐薬を入れておきます．後で薬が溶け出しておりものが増えるかもしれませんが，心配ありませんよ．

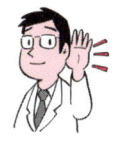

Listening comprehension

123. What is the patient's complaint?

（解答は別冊）

PART 1 整形外科

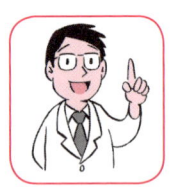

パターン1
〜する時，〜（部位）が〜の状態ですか

Are (is) 部位 + 状態 + when 〜?

例　Are your fingers painful + when you bend them?　指を曲げると痛みますか．

あてはめましょう！

a, b にそれぞれ下記の単語を組み合わせてみましょう．

Are (Is) [a] [b] ?

a) your hands 手, your extremities 四肢, your knees 膝, your ankles 足首, your shoulders 肩, your joints 関節
b) swollen 腫れる, numb 痺れる, weak 力が入らない, stiff こわばる

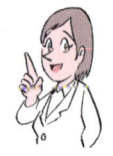

使えるパターンを増やそう！
〜すると痛いですか（特に部位を特定しない場合）

Is it painful + when 〜?

例　Is it painful when you turn over in bed?
　　寝返りすると / 痛いですか．→寝返りする時，痛いですか．

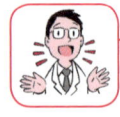

練習　このパターンでこれだけ話せる！（解答は別冊）

ヒント　日本文を英文に変換するとき，以下のように言い換えます．
124. 寝返りが / 痛いですか→寝返りをする時，痛いですか．
125. 歩き始めると / 痛いですか / →歩き始めた時，〜
126. 立ったり座ったりが / 痛いですか．→立ったり座ったりする時，〜
127. 階段の上がりが，/ 痛いですか．→階段を上がる時，〜
128. お尻から太ももにかけて /(部位)痛いですか．

整形外科

▶検査などでよく使う動作例

● Back Exam 背中の検査
I'll need to push all along your back. 背中に沿って押していきます.

●動きの範囲：
Can you bend down and touch your toes?　体を曲げると足の親指に届きますか.
Can you bend your knees back and forth?　膝を屈伸できますか.

●脚の筋肉の検査
Kick out. 蹴ってください.
Pull back. 後ろにひっぱってください.
Step on the gas. アクセルを踏んでください.
Pull up. 上にひっぱってあげてください.

●膝の反射など足の検査をする
Now, I'll tap to check your legs. 足をトントンします.
I'll tap the reflexes in your knees and ankles. 膝とくるぶしを軽くたたいて反射を調べます.
I'll need to push on the bottom of your legs. It may tickle a little. 足の裏を押します．少しくすぐったいですよ.
I'm going to check the good knee first. まず，状態が良い方の膝を調べます.
I'll push on your kneecap. 膝小僧を押します.
I'll touch your legs lightly. Do you feel that? 足を軽く触ります．わかりますか.
I need to see you walk. Can you walk across the room?　歩いているところを見ます．部屋の反対側の隅まで歩けますか.

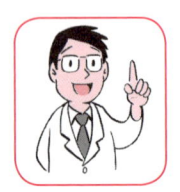

パターン2
〜すると(〜する時), 悪化しますか

Does the problem get worse ＋ when you 〜?

例　Does the problem get worse ＋ when you turn over in bed?
　　寝返りをすると, ひどくなりますか　→寝返りをする時, ひどくなりますか.

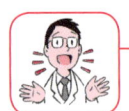

練習　このパターンでこれだけ話せる！　(解答は別冊)

129. 曲げると, 痛みがひどくなりますか.
130. 歩きまわると, 腫れがひどくなりますか.

words & expressions

align the bone in it's appropriate position, called reduction(整復)する
Please move your neck back and forth. 頸を / 前後に動かして
　－raise your shoulders 肩を / 挙げてみて
　－show me your palms 手のひらを / 見せて
　－clasp and unclasp your hands グーパーをして
　－bend your thumbs 親指を / 曲げてみて
　－bend and stretch your knees 膝を / 曲げて伸ばして
　－lie down on your back(/face) 診察台に仰向け(うつぶせに寝て)
　－bend your toes back 足の親指を / 反らして
　－bend backwards at the waist 腰を / 反らして
　－keep your back straight 背すじを伸ばして

整形外科

パターン3
～できますか
Can you ～?

例　Can you turn your head sideways?　頸をまわせますか.

あてはめましょう!

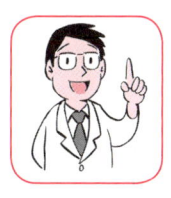

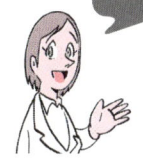

次の枠内に下記の用語をあてはめて，症状を尋ねてください．

Can you _____ ?

raise your shoulders 肩を挙げる，look up and look down 上を見たり下を見たり，stay sitting down 座る，squat down しゃがむ，stretch your back 腰を伸ばす，bend at the waist 腰を曲げる

用語・用法研究　When と while の使い分け

Q1．次の英文の違いは何ですか．
(1) Do you have any pain when walking?
(2) Do you have any pain while walking?
A1．実際の会話ではほぼ同じように使われます．異なる場合もありますが，ここは同じです．

Q2．次の英文の違いは？
(1) Is it painful when you start walking?
(2) Do you have any pain when you start walking?
(3) Do you have any pain when start walking?
A2．(3)は文法的に間違っています．when starting walking なら文法は大丈夫です．
Is it painful when you start walking?　の方が自然なようですが，Is it painful when starting walking? でも構いません．また，Do you have any pain in your back when you start walking? は自然です．Is it painful という表現は，一般的に痛みがあるのかという質問ですから，痛みの場所や本質について聞けません．

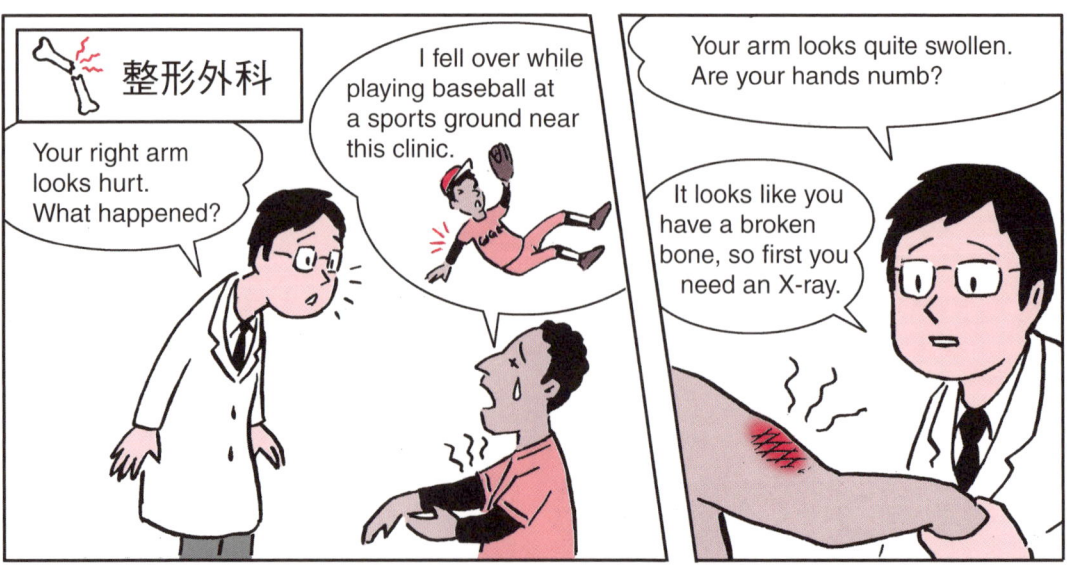

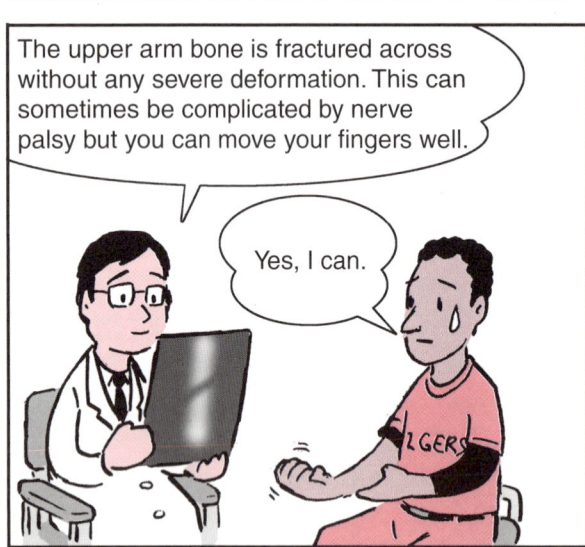

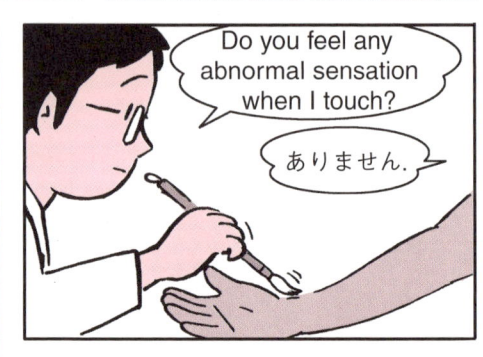

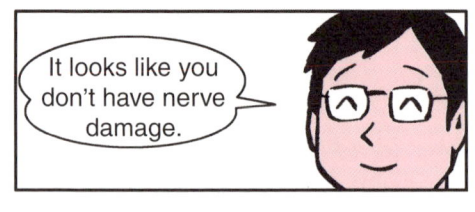

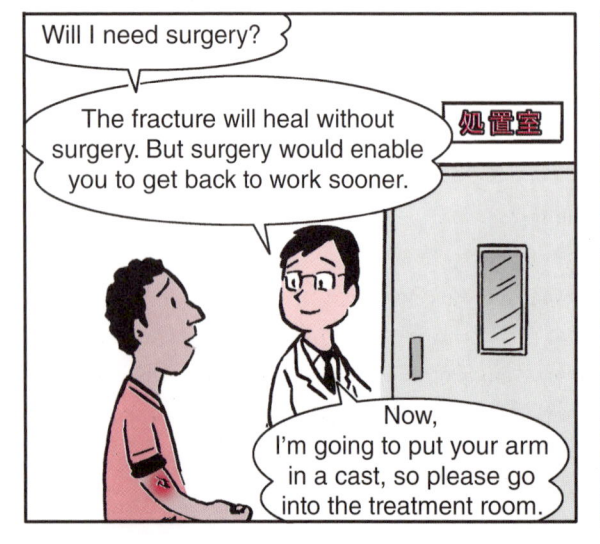

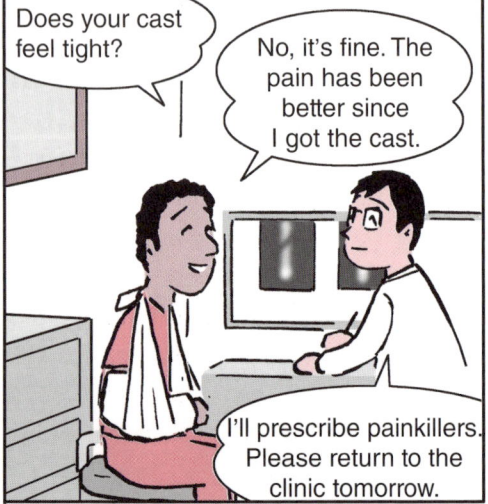

Case 14　上腕骨骨折（20歳男性）

〔*A patient enters the consultation room, cradling his right arm*〕

Dr. Your right arm looks hurt. What happened?

Pt. I fell over while playing baseball at a sports ground near this clinic.

Dr. Your arm looks quite swollen. Are your hands numb?

Pt. No, they aren't numb. But the pain is so terrible that I cannot stand it.

Dr. It looks like you have a broken bone, so first you need an X-ray.

〔*The doctor, while looking at the X-ray image*〕

Dr. The upper arm bone is fractured across without any severe deformation. This can sometimes be complicated by nerve palsy, but you can move your fingers well, can't you?

Pt. Yes, I can.

〔*The doctor talks, while touching around his thumb with a brush*〕

Dr. Do you feel any abnormal sensation?

Pt. No, I don't.

Dr. It looks like you don't have nerve damage (neuropathy).

Pt. That's a relief. Will I still need surgery?

Dr. The fracture will heal with a cast, without surgery. But surgery is preferable, because it would enable you to get back to work sooner.

Pt. In that case, what kind of surgery should I have?

Dr. There are several kinds of surgery, each of which has its advantages. We can discuss that later. If you don't have any other serious health problems, I recommend that you have surgery.

Pt. I understand. Let me give it some thought. I would like to talk about it with my family.

Dr. Now I'm going to put your arm in a cast, so please go into the treatment room.

〔*Putting the arm in a cast with a sling*〕

Does your cast feel tight?

Pt. No, it's fine. The pain has been better since I got the cast.

Dr. I'll prescribe painkillers. Please return to the clinic tomorrow.

〔右上腕を押さえて診察室に入ってくる〕
Dr. 右腕が痛そうですが，どうされましたか．
Pt. 近くのグラウンドで野球をしていて，転びました．
Dr. だいぶ腫れが強いですが，手が痺れたりはしていませんか．
Pt. 痺れはありませんが，痛くて我慢できません．
Dr. 骨折していると思われますので，まずレントゲン検査をします．
〔レントゲンを示しながら〕上腕骨が斜めに折れていますが，変形はひどくありません．神経麻痺を合併することがありますが，手の指はよく動きますね．
Pt. はい．ちゃんと動きます．
Dr. 〔箏を使って，親指あたりをさわり〕さわった感覚に異常はありませんか．
Pt. ありません．
Dr. 神経損傷は無いようですね．
Pt. それはよかった．でも，手術が必要ですか．
Dr. 手術をしなくても，ギプス固定で骨折は治りますが，手術をしたほうが，社会復帰は早くなります．
Pt. 手術を受けるとしたら，どういう手術になるのですか．
Dr. いろいろな手術法がありますが，それぞれ利点がありますので，追って検討することになります．ほかに大きな病気がないようでしたら，手術をすることをお勧めします．
Pt. わかりました．家族と相談して，少し考えてみます．
Dr. まず，ギプス固定をしますので，処置室にお入りください．〔ギプス固定を終えて〕ギプスはきつくないですか．
Pt. はい，大丈夫です．固定したら，痛みが楽になりました．
Dr. 鎮痛剤を処方しますので，明日また来院してください．

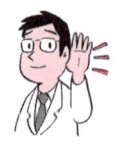

Listening comprehension

（解答は別冊）

131. Please choose the correct one.
    A. He has a transverse fracture with neuropathy
    B. He has a fracture in his lower arm（in his forearm）.
    C. The doctor recommended surgery.

Case 15-1　腰椎椎間板ヘルニア（32歳男性）

Dr. Sorry for keeping you waiting. What is the problem?

Pt. I've been suffering from severe pain and numbness around the outside of my left thigh for about a week. I've been waiting to see how it went, but it hasn't healed on its own. So, I came to see you.

Dr. When does it hurt?

Pt. It hurts most when working at my desk.

Dr. How do you feel while walking?

Pt. I feel better while walking.

Dr. How about while sleeping?

Pt. I feel much better when lying down.

Dr. Do you have any lower back pain?

Pt. No, not much.

Dr. Alright, please lie down on your back.

〔*The doctor notes the physical findings*〕

Dr. A positive leg raising test and hallux weakness (hyposthenia of the hallux) suggest that you may have sciatica due to lumbar disc hernia. I need to take an X-ray of your lower back. Is that OK with you?

Pt. Sure.

Dr. お待たせいたしました．どうされましたか．
Pt. 1週間前から，左太ももから足の外側にかけて，痺れと痛みがひどいのです．様子を見ていましたが，自然に治らないので来ました．
Dr. どういうときに痛みが起きますか．
Pt. 主に，デスクワークがつらいのです．
Dr. 歩くときはどうですか．
Pt. むしろ，歩いている時のほうが楽です．
Dr. 寝ているときはどうですか．
Pt. 横になっていれば，楽です．
Dr. 腰の痛みはありますか．
Pt. 腰痛はあまりありません．
Dr. では，こちらに（診察台に）仰向けになってください．
〔*理学所見をとる*〕
Dr. 足の挙上試験が陽性で，左拇趾の脱力があるので，腰椎椎間板ヘルニアによる坐骨神経痛が生じているようです．腰のレントゲン検査を受けていただきますが，よろしいですか．
Pt. わかりました．

Case 15-2 腰椎椎間板ヘルニア(32歳男性)

[*After the Xray*]

- Pt. What were the results?
- Dr. The X-ray shows a narrowed space between lumbar vertebrae four and five.
  The disc around here is protruding and pressing on a nerve. This is called a disc hernia, and causes pain radiating into the lower extremities.
- Pt. What should I do?
- Dr. You need bed rest and to take an antiphlogistic analgesic agent and a muscle relaxant for a week.
- Pt. I cannot take time off from my job.(I can't get a break from my job.)
- Dr. I'll give you a corset. Please put it on before going to work.
- Pt. Can I take baths?
- Dr. Yes, of course you can. In fact, baths will do you good.
- Pt. Do I need surgery?
- Dr. You don't need surgery for this problem. In most cases, the problem should be managed conservatively.
- Pt. I see. I'll take the drugs for a week, then.

〔レントゲン検査の後〕
- Pt. 結果はどうでしたか.
- Dr. 第4腰椎と第5腰椎の間が狭くなっています. この場所の椎間板が飛び出て, 神経を圧迫しているものと思われます. これを, 椎間板ヘルニアといい, 下肢に放散する痛みが生じます.
- Pt. どうすればよいのでしょうか.
- Dr. 安静にして, 消炎鎮痛剤と筋弛緩剤を1週間飲んでみてください.
- Pt. 仕事は休めないのですが.
- Dr. コルセットを処方しますので, 仕事に行く前にそれをつけてください.
- Pt. お風呂は入ってよいですか.
- Dr. むしろ, 入浴は効果的です.
- Pt. 手術になることはないですか.
- Dr. 今の症状ですと, 手術の適応はありません. 多くの場合は, 保存的治療で治癒します.
- Pt. わかりました. 1週間薬を飲んでみます.

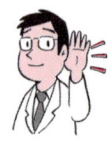

Listening comprehension （解答は別冊）

132. What is the most likely diagnosis?
133. Does he need surgery?

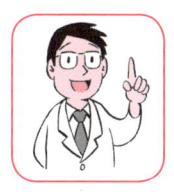

整形外科

パターン 4
診察時の会話

1. Let's do a test first, and then I 〜
   まず，検査をし，それから〜をしましょう．
2. The test shows 原因, so you (may) have 診断
   検査では(原因)が見られますので，(診断)でしょう．

   The test shows you (may) have 診断
   検査から(診断)であることがわかります．

例 1　Let's do a test. And then we can discuss the treatment plan.
　　　まず，検査を行って，それから治療方針を立てましょう．

例 2　The test shows disc degeneration, so you may have lower back pain.
　　　検査から椎間板変形がみられ，腰痛があると考えられます．

あてはめましょう！

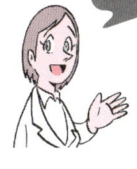

枠内に下記の a, b, c の言葉をそれぞれあてはめましょう

Let's do a test first, and then I [a] .

a) will look at the result and decide the best treatment. 結果をみて，最善の治療を決めましょう．
   will see if you need surgery. 手術が必要かどうか決めましょう．

The test [b] **you (may) have** [c] .

b) reveals, indicates, suggests, demonstrates 示します
c) a sprain 捻挫，a fracture 骨折，a stiff neck 首のコリ

109

Case 16-1 骨粗鬆症（75歳女性）

Pt. Hello, what were the test results?

Dr. The DEXA bone scan and the NTX urine test show that your bone density is much lower than average, so you may have osteoporosis.

Pt. What should I do?

Dr. You need to take care of yourself, including adopting a regular life-style, doing moderate exercise, and sun bathing. (You must try to adopt a regular life-style. This includes moderate exercise and sun exposure.) As for your diet, I'll give you a pamphlet about healthy eating, so please read through it.

Pt. Don't I need (to take) any medicine?

Dr. No, you don't. However, there are drugs called bisphosphonates for this. You are now receiving treatment for gum disease (periodentitis), aren't you?

Pt. Would that cause any problems?

Dr. Bisphosphonates have a rare side effect called jaw osteonecrosis. (This typically occurs) in those with gum disease and those who've had a recent dental procedure, such as a tooth extraction.
It is an effective medicine for osteoporosis, so I want to look into prescribing it after your dental treatment has finished.

Pt. I see.

Pt. こんにちは．検査の結果はいかがでしたか．

Dr. DEXA 骨スキャン，尿中 NTX の結果を見ると，あなたの骨密度は年齢よりだいぶ低いようですので，骨粗鬆症といえます．

Pt. どうしたらよろしいのでしょうか．

Dr. 規則正しい生活，適度な運動，それに日光浴も必要ですね．食事に関しては，パンフレットをお渡ししますので参考にしてください．

Pt. 薬は飲まなくてもよいのですか．

Dr. いいえ．実はビスホスホネートという薬があるのですが，あなたは今歯周炎で歯科治療中ですね．

Pt. それが，なにか影響あるのですか．

Dr. 頻度は少ないのですが，ビスホスホネートには顎骨壊死という副作用があって，歯周炎があるときや抜歯などの歯科的処置を受けるとその副作用を起こすことがあります．骨粗鬆症にはとてもよい薬なので，歯科治療が終わってから処方を検討したいと思います．

Pt. わかりました．

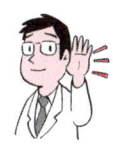

Listening comprehension

（解答は別冊）

134. Please choose the correct one.
   A. She is given bisphonate for osteonecrosis.
   B. She needs to consult with a dentist for osteonecrosis.
   C. She is not given bisphonate, because she is now receiving dental treatment.

Case 16-2   骨粗鬆症（75歳女性）

[*At the dental office*]

Dr. Hello, is it true that you are going to be taking osteoporosis drugs?

Pt. Yes, I am.

Dr. Recently, the causal relationship between the use of osteoporosis drugs and jaw osteonecrosis has become controversial. Current opinion is that the use of oral osteoporosis drugs doesn't increase the risk of osteonecrosis of the jaw as a complication of ordinary dental procedures. (The use of oral osteoporosis drugs doesn't have harmful effects on the jawbones as a complication of ordinary dental procedures).

Pt. I see.

Dr. But when treating a patient who is on IV osteoporosis drugs or who needs to have a tooth extracted, we contact their physician and, if necessary, the osteoporosis drugs are temporarily discontinued.

Pt. I understand.

Dr. In your case, you have rather advanced periodontal disease, so I recommend regular dental cleaning and oral exams to prevent further disease progression. Controlling gum disease can also help with the management of other health problems, such as chronic inflammatory conditions.

Pt. What are the causes of this disease?

Dr. You don't need to worry about it; 80% of Japanese suffer from gum disease. Natural changes in the gums occur to some degree as you age, as with the rest of the body. It is also closely related to other health problems. We'll have to keep a watchful eye on your gums.

Pt. Yes, thank you. How often should I come?

Dr. I'll give you a specific recommendation once I've examined your mouth, but in general you should come about once every four months.

整形外科

〔歯科医院にて〕

Dr. こんにちは．骨粗鬆症のお薬を服用されることになったのですね．
Pt. はい．
Dr. 最近は，顎骨壊死について騒がれていますが，経口投与の場合は，通常の歯科治療は差し支えないといわれています．
Pt. そうでしたか．
Dr. ただ，お薬を静注投与したり，歯を抜かなければならなくなったときには，お薬を処方された先生と連携をとり，一時的にお薬の服用を中止することもあります．
Pt. わかりました．
Dr. あなたの場合は，歯周病がやや進んでいるため，定期的なクリーニングと口腔内のチェックをし，歯周病の進行を和らげることをおすすめします．歯周病のコントロールをすると慢性疾患など他の全身の病気のケアにもつながりますよ．
Pt. どうして，こんなふうになってしまったのでしょう．
Dr. そんなに心配なさらなくても，日本人の8割が歯周病にかかっているといわれています．歯周病も体の他の部位と一緒で，加齢とともに増えていきます．また，歯周病は他の健康障害にも密接に関係しています．ですから，上手に歯周病とお付き合いしていきましょう．
Pt. お願いします．どのくらいのペースで来たらよいですか．
Dr. 口腔内の状態をみてこちらから指示いたしますが，だいたい4ヵ月に1度と考えておいてください．

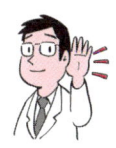

Listening comprehension （解答は別冊）

Please write false (F) or true (T).

The dentist told the patient that

135. osteoporosis drugs should be temporarily discontinued. (　　)
136. controlling gum disease is related to the management of other health problems. (　　)

Coffee break

ビスホスホネートは，経口投与では副反応がないと断言できるエビデンスはまだありません．ビスホスホネートに関しての日本でのデータは，まだ使用例が少ないため正確にはわからないのです．ただ，通常の歯科治療では，抜歯以外に顎骨壊死等を起こすような状況になることは考えにくいとされています．従って，ビスホスホネートを服用しているからという理由で歯科治療を控えることにより，歯科的な悪化をきたすと考えられる場合は，むしろ治療を優先した方が良いでしょう．

パターン5 指示

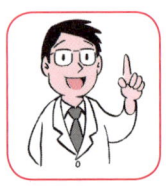

1 Please get bed rest.　絶対安静にしてください.
2 Please take time off work.　仕事を休んでください.
3 Please take gentle exercise.　軽い運動をしてください.
4 Please change your own dressing.　自分でガーゼを交換してください.
5 Please don't take baths.　お風呂に入らないでください.
6 Please don't walk long distances.　長い間歩かないでください.
7 Please come back here frequently for follow-up.
経過観察のためにまめにきてください.
8 Please make an appointment for your next visit.
次の診察(検査)の予約を取ってください.

用語・用法研究　Apply, Give, Perform の使い分け

① Apply の使用例

Apply a cast, so the bones will be immobilized.　骨がずれないように，ギプスをつけましょう.
　　– tape directly over the dressings on the wound.　傷口の包帯の上に直接テープををつけてください.
　　– cream and ointment.　クリームと軟膏をぬってください.
　　– a poultice wound dressing.　湿布を使ってください.

② Give の使用例

Give an intraarticular injection.　関節に注射をしましょう.
　　– medications(drugs).　薬をあげましょう.
　　– vaccination.　ワクチンをあげましょう.

③ Perform の使用例

Perform physical therapy.
　　– surgery.　手術をします.
　　– conservative therapy(preservative therapy).　保存的治療をします.

④ Do の使用例

Do a test.　検査をします.
　　– a culture and stain.　培養と染色をします.
　　– a bone biopsy.　骨生検をします.
　　– a diagnostic procedure.　確定診断をします.

Case 17　手根管症候群（24 歳女性）

- Dr. What brings you in today?
- Pt. I am now seven months pregnant, and I've been suffering from numbness in my right hand for 2 months. I am having difficulty using my hand.
- Dr. Which part of your hand?
- Pt. Around my index finger and middle finger.
- Dr. Please show me your right hand. The ball of your thumb has shrunk, so I imagine it's difficult to pick up small change, right?
- Pt. Yes.

   〔*Describing physical findings including Tinel sign and Fahren's Test*〕

- Dr. The range of the numbness and physical findings indicate that you most likely have carpal tunnel syndrome. Does it hurt?
- Pt. It is not painful, but the numbness gets intense around dawn. It sometimes wakes me up.
- Dr. That is one of the characteristics of this disease.
   Now you need to take a nerve conduction test to confirm the diagnosis.
- Pt. I see. What sort of disease is it?
- Dr. The causes of this disease are unknown in many cases, but it tends to develop more often in women than in men. It is most likely to develop during pregnancy. Carpal tunnel syndrome is a condition in which the nerve called the median nerve passing through the carpal tunnel in the wrist is compressed. The treatment for it can include oral drugs, resting the wrist, injections, and surgery, but sometimes it gets better on its own. In your case, you are pregnant, so I would like to see how things go if you just use a hand brace during the night. Is that OK with you?
- Pt. Yes, please.
- Dr. After you make an appointment for the test, I'll show you to the treatment room.

Dr. どうされましたか
Pt. 妊娠7ヵ月なのですが，この2ヵ月間右手がしびれて使いにくいのです．
Dr. 手のどの辺りですか．
Pt. 人差し指と中指あたりです．
Dr. それでは，右手を見せてください．親指の付け根のふくらみが小さくなっていますね．これだと，小銭がつまみにくいでしょう．
Pt. はい．
〔*Tinel sign, Fahren's Test* などの理学所見をとる〕
Dr. しびれの範囲や理学所見から見ると，手根管症候群という病気がもっとも考えられます．痛みはありますか．
Pt. 痛みはありませんが，明け方などしびれが強くなって起きてしまうことがあります．
Dr. それも，この病気の特徴のひとつです．まず，診断を確定するために神経伝導速度の測定という検査を受けていただきます．
Pt. わかりました．その病気はどのような病気ですか．
Dr. 多くは原因不明ですが，圧倒的に女性に多く生じます．
妊婦に起こることも多いです．正中神経という神経が手首にある手根管というトンネルの中で圧迫されている状態です．治療は飲み薬，手首の安静，注射，手術などがありますが，自然と治ることも多くみられます．あなたの場合は，妊娠中ということもありますので，夜間装具で経過を見させていただいてよろしいでしょうか．
Pt. わかりました．
Dr. それでは，検査の予約をお取りになった後，処置室にご案内いたします．

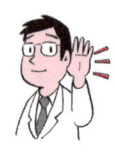

Listening comprehension (解答は別冊)

137. What is the most likely diagnosis?
138. What kinds of test does she need to take to confirm the diagnosis?

PART 1

皮膚科

パターン1 問診例

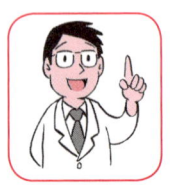

1. How can I help you?　どうしましたか.

2. Where do you feel itchy? Your whole body?
   どこがかゆいですか. 身体中ですか.
   Does the area feel itchy?　そこはかゆいですか.

3. What is it like? Itchy? Or painfully itchy?
   どんなかゆみですか. むずがゆいですか, 痛がゆいですか.
   （ヒント）英語でむずがゆいに当たる言葉はない.

4. When do you feel itchy? For example, is it all the time? At night (when asleep)?　いつかゆいですか. 1日中ですか, 夜間（睡眠時）ですか.

5. How bad is it? Does the itching keep you awake?
   どの程度ですか. かゆくて眠れませんか.

6. Have you noticed a rash?　発疹に気づいていますか.

7. Have you felt itchy before?　これまでかゆいことがありましたか.

words & expressions

a swelling できもの（はれもの）, a rash 発疹, a pimple にきび, a wart イボ, a tumor 腫瘍, an abscess 膿, a blister 膿疱
itchy かゆい, むずがゆい, むずむずする, pus-filled 膿が詰まった
dry かさかさの, chapped 肌荒れの, puffy 腫れた, irritated ヒリヒリする, crusty かさぶた状の, burning sensation 焼けるような感覚
pricking pain チクチクする痛み, piercing pain/boring pain/crampy pain 差し込むような痛み, smarting pain/stinging pain ヒリヒリする痛み
pin-prick sensation 針で刺すような痛み, throbbing pain ズキズキする痛み
gripping pain 締め付けるような痛み, shooting pain つきぬけるような痛み

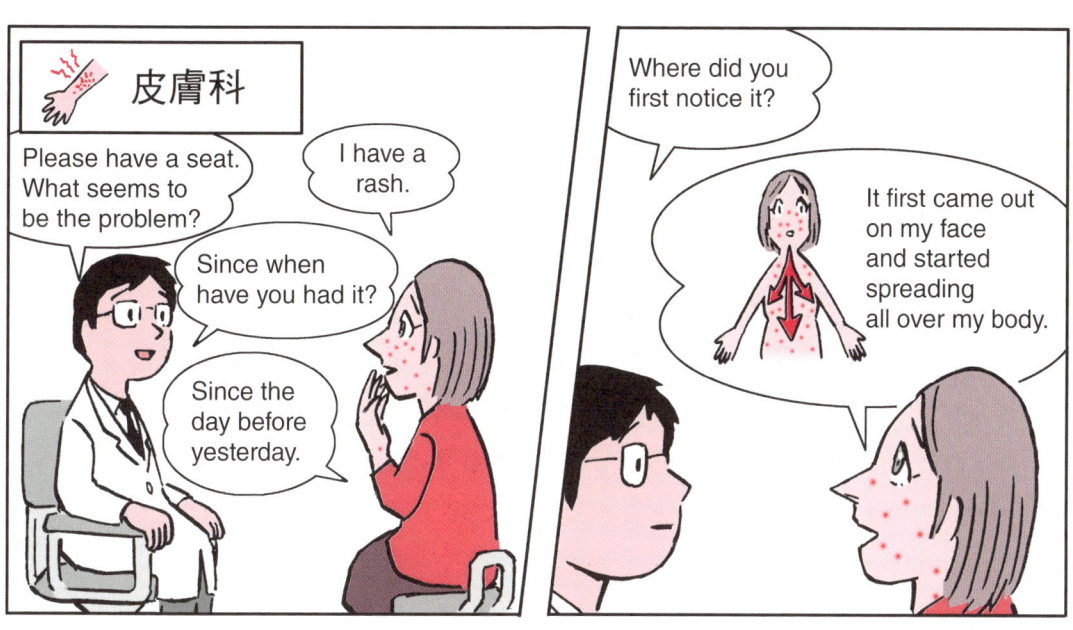

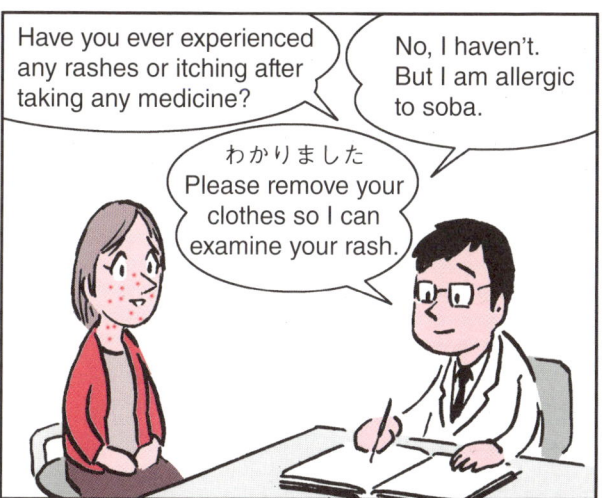

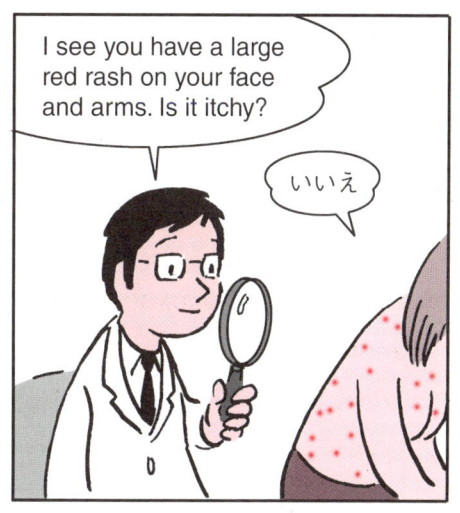

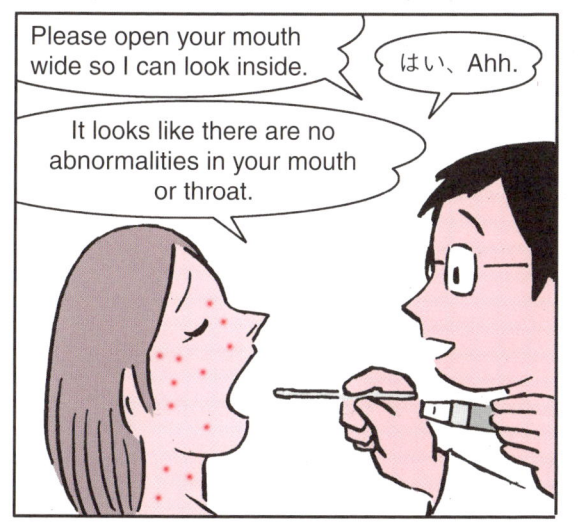

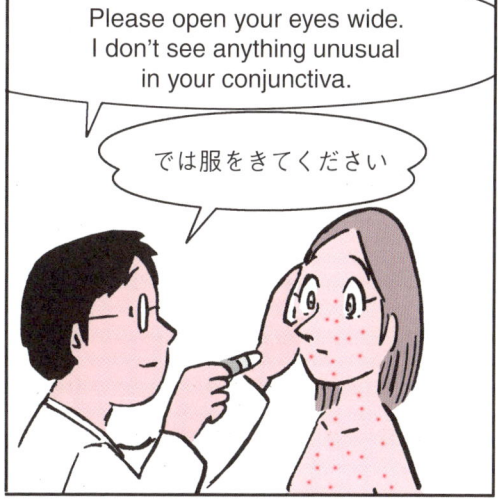

皮膚科

皮膚科

Please have a seat. What seems to be the problem?

I have a rash.

Since when have you had it?

Since the day before yesterday.

Where did you first notice it?

It first came out on my face and started spreading all over my body.

Have you ever experienced any rashes or itching after taking any medicine?

No, I haven't. But I am allergic to soba.

わかりました Please remove your clothes so I can examine your rash.

I see you have a large red rash on your face and arms. Is it itchy?

いいえ

Please open your mouth wide so I can look inside.

はい、Ahh.

It looks like there are no abnormalities in your mouth or throat.

Please open your eyes wide. I don't see anything unusual in your conjunctiva.

では服をきてください

119

Case 18-1 薬剤アレルギー（薬疹）（50歳男性）

- Dr. Hello, please have a seat. What seems to be the problem?
- Pt. I have a rash.
- Dr. Since when have you had it?
- Pt. Since the day before yesterday.
- Dr. Where did you first notice it?
- Pt. It first came out on my face and started spreading all over my body.
- Dr. Do you have any other health problems at the moment?
- Pt. I have been told I have high blood pressure.
- Dr. Are you currently taking any medicine?
- Pt. Yes, this.

    〔*The patient shows a medication prescription.*〕

- Dr. Have you changed your medication recently?
- Pt. My blood pressure didn't go down, so I was prescribed an additional drug.
- Dr. When did you start the new one?
- Pt. One week ago.
- Dr. Have you ever experienced any rashes or itching after taking any medicine?
- Pt. No, I haven't. But I am allergic to soba.

    ****

- Dr. Please remove your clothes so I may examine your rash. I see you have a large red rash on your face and body. Is it itchy?
- Pt. No.
- Dr. Please open your mouth wide so I may look inside.
- Pt. Certainly, Ahh〔*opening his mouth*〕.
- Dr. It looks like there are no (mucosal) abnormalities in your mouth or throat. Do you have a sore throat?
- Pt. No.
- Dr. Do you have any other symptoms aside from the rash, such as a fever?
- Pt. No. Nothing in particular.

皮膚科

Dr. Now please open your eyes wide. I don't see any (conjunctival) abnormalities.

Dr.	こんにちは．おかけください．今日はどうなさいましたか．	Pt.	いいえ．お薬で出たことはありません．でも，ソバアレルギーがあります．
Pt.	発疹が出ているのですが．		********************
Dr.	いつからですか．	Dr.	わかりました．では，服を脱いで，発疹をみせてください．顔，体に赤い発疹がたくさんみられますね．かゆみがありますか．
Pt.	2日前からです．		
Dr.	最初，どこに気がつきましたか．		
Pt.	最初，顔に出て，体にひろがってきています．	Pt.	いいえ．
Dr.	現在，ほかの病気はありませんか．	Dr.	では，大きく口をあけて，口の中をみせてください．
Pt.	高血圧症といわれています．		
Dr.	お薬は飲んでいますか．	Pt.	はい．あ〜〔口を開けながら〕．
Pt.	はい，これです．〔薬剤情報書をみせながら〕	Dr.	口の粘膜，のどには異常はないようです．のどが痛みますか．
Dr.	最近，お薬がかわりましたか．		
Pt.	血圧が下がらないので，1つ追加になりました．	Pt.	いいえ．
		Dr.	現在，発疹以外に，熱があるとか，身体の調子が悪いところがありますか．
Dr.	いつ，追加されましたか．		
Pt.	1週間前に追加されました．	Pt.	特にありません．
Dr.	これまで，お薬を飲んで，蕁麻疹や発疹が出たことがありますか．	Dr.	次は，眼を大きく開いてください．結膜に異常はないようです．

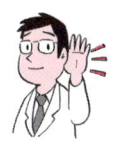

[Listening comprehension]　　　　　　　　　　　（解答は別冊）

139. What is the patient's chief complaint?　Please choose the correct one.
　　　A. fever　　B. rash　　C. soba allergy

Case 18-2　薬剤アレルギー（薬疹）（50歳男性）　CD2 trk 17-19

Dr. Looking at the rash, I suspect you have a drug rash.

Pt. What is a drug rash?

Dr. Drug rashes result from an allergic reaction to a drug.

Pt. I've never had one before. Is there any connection between that and my soba allergy?

Dr. No, it has no connection. Even if you have never had a drug rash before, you could still have one now.

Pt. What caused it?

121

Dr. It may have been caused by the blood pressure drug you started taking recently. I need to do a blood test.

Pt. What kind of test?

Dr. I'll take some of your blood to identify the cause of the rash. If the lymphocytes react with the medicine,(If there are certain types of cells in your blood,) we can assume that the medicine is the cause.

Pt. How long will it take to get the results?

Dr. It is a specific test, so it will take a week to get the result.

Pt. What should I do until then?

Dr. First of all, please stop taking the drug. If the drug causes the rash, it may then go away.

Pt. Is there anything else I should be concerned about?

Dr. If your condition doesn't improve after stopping the drug, please come back to see me.

Dr. 発疹からは薬疹が疑われます．
Pt. 薬疹ってなんですか．
Dr. お薬が合わなくて出てくる発疹のことです．
Pt. 今までそんなことはないのですが．ソバアレルギーと関係ありますか．
Dr. 今までなくても，薬疹が出ることはありえます．ソバアレルギーとは関連ありません．
Pt. 原因はなんでしょうか．
Dr. おそらく新たに追加された血圧の薬でしょう．血液検査をしましょう．
Pt. どのような検査をするのですか．
Dr. 採血して発疹の原因を特定しましょう．血液中のリンパ球がお薬と反応すれば（血中にある種の細胞があれば），その薬が原因と考えられます．
Pt. 結果はどれくらいで出ますか．
Dr. 特殊検査なので，結果がわかるのに1週間かかります．
Pt. それまでどうしたらいいですか．
Dr. まず，原因と思われるお薬を中止してみましょう．そのお薬が原因なら，発疹は消えてくると思います．
Pt. あと気をつけることはありますか．
Dr. 薬を中止したにもかかわらず症状が良くならなければ，すぐに受診してください．

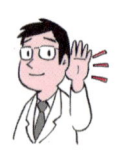

[Listening comprehension]

（解答は別冊）

140. What is the most likely diagnosis?
141. What are the doctor's instructions?

Case 19-1　アトピー性皮膚炎（22歳女性）

Dr. Hello, please have a seat. What's the problem today?

Pt. I've been feeling itchy.

Dr. Since when?

Pt. About one month ago, soon after it got cold. It is often worse in the winter months, and it is particularly bad this year.

Dr. Which parts of your body are affected?

Pt. All over.

Dr. When do you feel itchy?

Pt. At night.

Dr. How severe is it? Does the itching keep you awake at night?

Pt. Yes, I itch so much that I often wake up.

Dr. Have you ever suffered from allergic skin conditions?

Pt. Yes, I often had eczema when I was a child.

Dr. Do you have any other type of allergies, such as asthma, allergic rhinitis, or food allergies?

Pt. I have hay fever.

Dr. Do any of your relatives have allergies?

Pt. My mother has skin allergies that I know of.

Dr. Okay. Please let me see the affected areas.

Dr. こんにちは．おかけください．今日はどうなさいましたか．
Pt. かゆいのですが．
Dr. いつからですか．
Pt. 1ヵ月前からです．寒くなってからです．いつも冬になるとかゆくなります．今年は特にひどいです．
Dr. どこがかゆいのですか．
Pt. 身体中です．
Dr. いつかゆいですか．
Pt. かゆいのは夜です．
Dr. どれくらいひどいですか．かゆみが強くて眠れませんか．
Pt. かゆみで目がさめてしまいます．
Dr. これまで肌が弱い体質がありますか．
Pt. 小さい頃はよく湿疹が出ました．
Dr. 皮膚以外のアレルギー，たとえば喘息，アレルギー性鼻炎，食物アレルギーなどがありますか．
Pt. 花粉症があります．
Dr. 血のつながった人にアレルギーがありますか．
Pt. 母は皮膚が弱いようです．
Dr. わかりました．では，かゆいところをみせてください．

[Listening comprehension]　　　　　　(解答は別冊)

142. What is the patient's past medical history?　Please choose the correct one.
　　A.　hay fever　　B.　brachial asthma　　C.　eczema

Case 19-2　アトピー性皮膚炎（22歳女性）　CD2 trk 20

Dr. I see you have a strong red rash all over your face and around the eyes.
〔*Examining his eyes, the doctor says*〕
Your eyes appear injected. Is there anything unusual about your vision?

Pt. No, there isn't.

Dr. In that case, please undress and let me see the parts of your body where you feel itchy. I see you have dry skin, eczema and scratch marks on your back. Are there any other affected areas?

Pt. My arms and legs itch as well.

Dr. You also have rashes on the inside of your elbows and knees. Do you have any other problems or symptoms such as a fever?

Pt. No, nothing in particular.

Dr. OK, please put on your clothes.
〔diagnosis〕

Dr. I suspect your problem may be atopic dermatitis.

Pt. What causes it?

Dr. One of the causes is an inherited allergic skin. The skin condition is aggravated by dry air, and the air becomes very dry in winter.

Pt. Is it related to my hay fever?

Dr. Hay fever is also an allergic condition. Please let me do a blood test.

Pt. What kind of test is that?

Dr. I'll take some of your blood to assess an amount of an antibody called IgE, which is related to allergic reactions.

Pt. I see. In any case, could you do something about the itching?

Dr. Please take antihistamines twice a day, after breakfast and after your evening meal.

皮膚科

Pt. Will they make me sleepy?
Dr. I'll prescribe a drug that makes you less drowsy and an ointment.
Pt. When should I apply the ointment?
Dr. The best time to apply it is after you take a bath.
Pt. Is there anything else I should be aware of?
Dr. Please try to avoid scratching the affected areas.
Pt. Is there any food I should avoid?
Dr. Also please avoid spicy foods and alcohol, which can make the itching worse.

Dr. 顔全体と目の周囲に強い発赤がみられます．
〔服を診察しながら〕
Dr. 結膜が充血しています．視力の異常はありませんか．
Pt. 特にありません．
Dr. では，服を脱いで身体のかゆいところをみせてください．背中がかさかさですね．湿疹と掻き傷が混じっています．ほかにかゆいところがありますか．
Pt. 腕や脚がかゆいです．
Dr. 肘や膝の内側に湿疹がみられますね．現在，発疹以外に，熱があるとか，身体の調子が悪いところがありますか．
Pt. 特にありません．
Dr. では，服を着てください．
〔診断〕
Dr. 症状からはアトピー性皮膚炎が疑われます．
Pt. 原因はなんですか．
Dr. 遺伝的な皮膚の過敏体質です．冬になると空気が乾燥して悪化します．

Pt. 花粉症と関係ありますか．
Dr. 花粉症（アレルギー性鼻炎）もアレルギー疾患の一つです．血液検査をさせてください．
Pt. どのような検査をするのですか．
Dr. 採血して，血液中のIgEというアレルギーに関係している抗体の量を調べます．
Pt. わかりました．とにかく，かゆみを止めてください．
Dr. かゆみ止めの抗ヒスタミン薬を1日2回，朝食後と夕食後に服用してください．
Pt. 眠くなりませんか．
Dr. 眠気の少ない薬を処方しましょう．塗り薬も差し上げます．
Pt. 塗り薬はいつ塗るのですか．
Dr. 入浴後がベストです．
Pt. ほかに気をつけることはありますか．
Dr. できるだけ掻かないようにしてください．
Pt. 食事に気をつけることはありますか．
Dr. 辛い物やアルコールはかゆみを増しますから，控えてください．

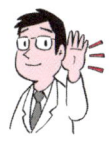

[Listening comprehension] （解答は別冊）

143. What is the most likely diagnosis?
144. What are the doctor's instructions?

coffee break

・かゆみと病気

皮膚は内臓の鏡といわれるように，内科疾患を反映してかゆみが起こることがあります．かゆみを訴えるにもかかわらず皮膚に発疹がない場合には，内科疾患を精査する必要があります．かゆみを起こす内科疾患としては，腎不全，肝硬変，糖尿病，甲状腺疾患が有名ですが，まれに膠原病や内臓・血液悪性腫瘍に由来することもあるので忘れてはなりません．

・爪と病気

爪の異常としては爪白癬が最も有名です．爪が直接真菌におかされて肥厚・白濁が起こります．そのほか，爪の異常は爪周囲または全身の皮膚病を反映して起こることがあります．また，爪の異常から内科疾患がみつかることもあります．爪の異常を伴う内科疾患としては，貧血，心疾患，肺疾患，肝・腎疾患が知られています．爪の異常をみたら，皮膚疾患のみならず，常に内科疾患の合併を念頭に置く必要があります．

PART 1 眼 科

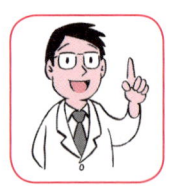

パターン 1

問診1　どちらが〜ですか
Which(one)〜

1 **Which is** more blurry, distant objects or near things like writing?
見えにくいのは，遠くですか．それとも近くの手元の文字ですか．

2 **Which is** itchy, your eye or your eyelids?
かゆいのは目の玉，それとも，まぶたですか．
Which one feels itchy?　どちらがかゆいですか．

3 **Which part is** irritated（uncomfortable），the surface or back of the eyes?
チクチク痛いのは，目の表面ですか．それとも目の奥ですか．

4 **Which eye** is painful, right or left, or are both painful?
痛みがあるのはどちらの目ですか．

Easy talk!　少し複雑な質問の対処方法

1　症状を尋ねた後
2　それはどこですか＋具体的な場所
を挙げると短い文で尋ねることができます．

例）ぴかぴか光る感じは中心ですか，周辺の端のほうですか．
⇒ぴかぴか光る感じはありますか，それはどこですか，中心ですか周辺の端のほうですか．

1　Do you see flashing lights?
2　Where do you see them, in the middle of the eye or in the peripheral field（at the edge）?

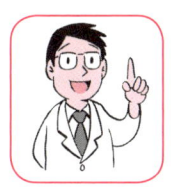

パターン2
問診2

1 飛蚊症について尋ねる

You see black spots or glare?
黒いものやまぶしい光が見えますか.

Do they move?　それはフワフワ動きますか.

Do they stay put (Are they fixed) in the center of the visual field (in front of your eyes)?　視野のまん中にとどまっていますか.

2 痛みについて尋ねる

Is it sometimes painful?　それは時々痛みますか.

When does the pain occur?　いつ痛みが起こったのですか.

How long does the pain last?　どのくらい続きましたか.

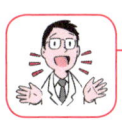

練習 このパターンでこれだけ話せる！ （解答は別冊）

145. 目が乾いた感じがしたりごろごろすれば，ドライアイの可能性があります.
146. 目がかすみますか．または，二重にみえることがありますか．涙がたくさん出ますか.
147. だぶって見えるのは，両目で見た時ですか，片目で見た時ですか.

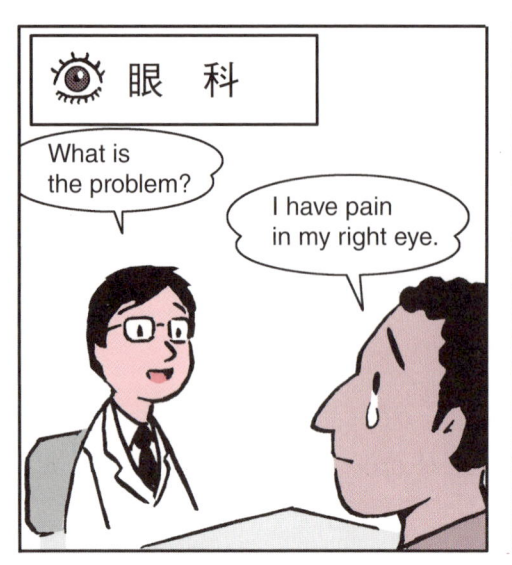

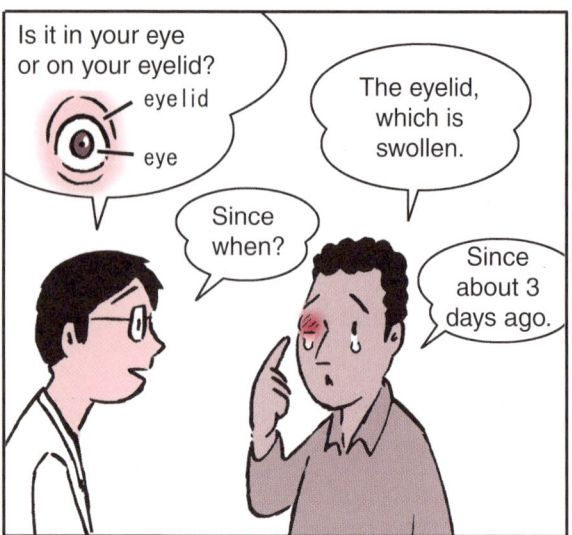

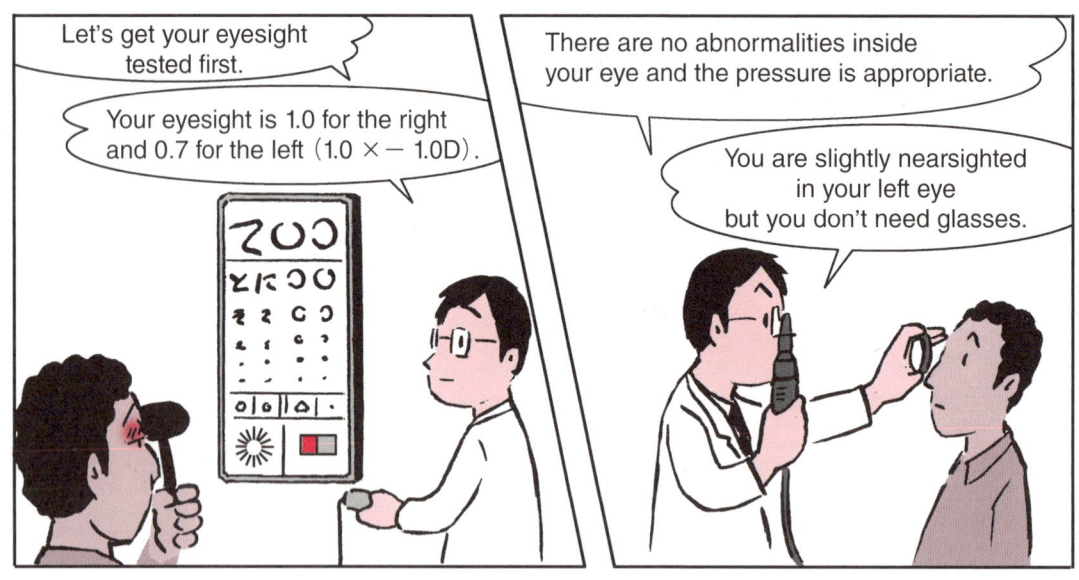

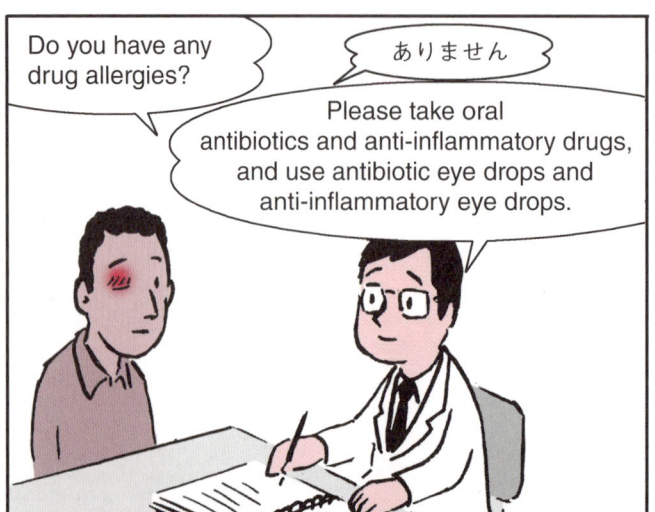

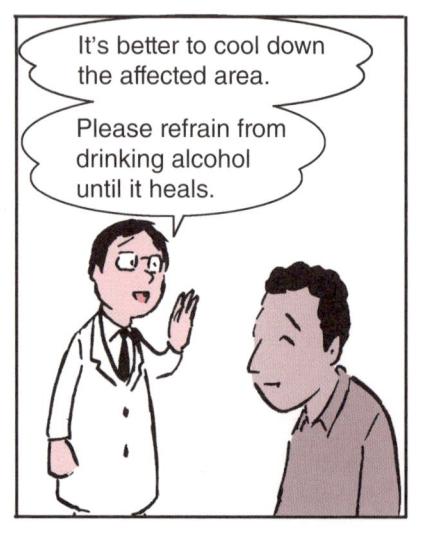

眼 科

What is the problem?

I have pain in my right eye.

Is it in your eye or on your eyelid?
- eyelid
- eye

The eyelid, which is swollen.

Since when?

Since about 3 days ago.

Let's get your eyesight tested first.

Your eyesight is 1.0 for the right and 0.7 for the left (1.0 × − 1.0D).

There are no abnormalities inside your eye and the pressure is appropriate.

You are slightly nearsighted in your left eye but you don't need glasses.

Do you have any drug allergies?

ありません

Please take oral antibiotics and anti-inflammatory drugs, and use antibiotic eye drops and anti-inflammatory eye drops.

It's better to cool down the affected area.

Please refrain from drinking alcohol until it heals.

Case 20　麦粒腫（30歳男性）

Dr. What is the problem?

Pt. I have pain in my right eye.

Dr. Is it in your eye or on your eyelid?

Pt. It is my eyelid. It's swollen.

Dr. Since when?

Pt. Since about 3 days ago.

Dr. Let's get your eyesight tested first. [*following test*] Your eyesight is 1.0 for the right eye and 0.7 for the left eye $(1.0 \times -1.0D)$. There are no abnormalities inside your eye and the pressure is appropriate. You are slightly nearsighted in your left eye, but you don't need glasses. Do you have any drug allergies?

Pt. No.

Dr. In that case, please take oral antibiotics and anti-inflammatory drugs, and use antibiotic eye drops and anti-inflammatory eye drops. It's better to cool down the affected area. Please refrain from drinking alcohol until it heals.

Dr.　どうしましたか．
Pt.　右目が痛いのです．
Dr.　痛いのは，眼球ですか，まぶたですか．
Pt.　まぶたです．上のまぶたが腫れまして．
Dr.　いつからですか．
Pt.　3日前からです．
Dr.　まず，視力を計りますね．[*検査後*] 視力は，右 = 1.0．左 = 0.7 [矯正 1.0 × (－1.0D)]．眼底，眼圧は両眼とも異常ありません．左の目に軽い近視がありますが，眼鏡は必要ないでしょう．お薬によるアレルギーはありませんか．
Pt.　ありません．
Dr.　それでは，抗生物質と消炎剤の点眼薬と内服薬とを用いてください．患部を少し冷やした方が良いですよ．お酒は治るまでやめてください．

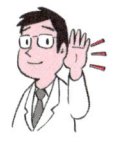

[Listening comprehension]　　　　（解答は別冊）

148. What is the most likely diagnosis?
149. What kinds of drugs are prescribed?

Case 21　角膜異物（40歳男性）

Dr. What is wrong with your eyes?
Pt While I was hammering a nail, something flew into my left eye and it hurts.
Dr. When did it happen?
Pt Just before, about one hour ago.
Dr. Let me examine your eyes. It appears as though you have a piece of metal stuck in your cornea. What is your profession?
Pt I'm a carpenter.
Dr. The object in your eye may be not a nail but a piece of metal equipment. I'll anesthetize it with eye drops.
Pt The pain has gone.
Dr. You aren't cured yet. I'm going to remove the foreign body from your cornea.
Pt What? Is there something stuck in the iris (and pupil) of my eye?
Dr. Yes, it is. It is in deep, but I'll get it all out if possible.
Pt How will you remove it?
Dr. （I'll remove it）with a fine needle. It won't hurt, so please hold still.
Pt No way! No!
Dr. I've got it. It was almost all the way through the cornea. If it had gone through the cornea, it would have been really serious.
Pt I feel so much better.
Dr. The anesthetic is still working. Afterward, I'll give you eye drops and medicine to take. Please come back tomorrow.

Dr. どうしましたか．
Pt. 釘を打っている時に，何かが左目に入り，痛みます．
Dr. いつですか．
Pt. 少し前で，1時間ほど前です．
Dr. 診てみましょう．角膜に鉄の破片が刺さっていますよ．お仕事は何ですか．
Pt. 大工です．

Dr. 刺さっているのはおそらく，釘の破片ではなく，金鎚の破片でしょう．点眼薬で麻酔をします．
Pt. 楽になりました．
Dr. 治ったわけではありませんよ．今から黒目の異物を取ります．
Pt. えっ！黒目に刺さっていますか．
Dr. そう．黒目にささっています．深いですが，

眼　科

出来るだけ全部取ります．
Pt. どうやって，取るのですか．
Dr. 細い針のようなモノで取ります．痛くないですから，動かないでください．
Pt. あ〜こわいです．
Dr. 取れました．ほとんど角膜の全層に刺さっていました．もし，角膜を貫通していたなら大変なことだったのですよ．
Pt. 楽になりました．
Dr. いまは麻酔が効いているからです．あとは，目薬と内服薬を出します．また明日来てください．

（注）職人の鎚が使いこまれたため，鎚の破片が飛んだ症例．

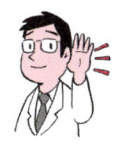

[Listening comprehension]　　　　　　　　　　（解答は別冊）

150. What is the most likely diagnosis?
151. What was the treatment?

Case 22　網膜剥離（30歳女性）

Dr. What is the trouble?

Pt. Suddenly, my vision has become blurred and I have difficulty seeing.

Dr. Since when?

Pt. Since yesterday.

Dr. Your visual acuity is $0.3 (0.4 \times -0.75D)$ for the right eye and 1.0 for the left. I'll perform a fundus oculi examination. Have you noticed any change in your eyes recently?

Pt. Now you mention it, I've been seeing some things like black specks floating around for about 7 days.

Dr. I think that was a warning sign. Your problem is a detached retina. A hole has opened in the retina, and part of it has peeled partially away. You need to be admitted to a well-equipped hospital for surgery.

Pt. What if I leave it, without having surgery?

Dr. Unfortunately, if it's left untreated you'll lose your sight. I'll arrange to have you admitted to the hospital. Please go as soon as possible. Until then, please refrain from strenuous exercise, which will make it worse.

Dr. どうしましたか.
Pt. 目が急にかすんで，見えにくくなりました.
Dr. いつからですか.
Pt. 昨日からです.
Dr. 視力は，右 = 0.3 (0.4×(-0.75D). 左 = 1.0. 眼底検査を致します．前から，変わったことは無かったでしょうか.
Pt. そういえば，7日前ごろから，黒いモノが飛んでいる様に見えていました.
Dr. それは，前兆だったのでしょうね．病気は，網膜剥離です．目の中の網膜に穴が開いて，網膜の一部が部分的に剥がれています．設備の整った病院に入院して手術を受ける必要があります.
Pt. 手術をせずにいると，どうなりますか.
Dr. 残念ながら，放置すると失明に至ります．入院のための病院を紹介いたしますから，できるだけ早く行ってください．激しい運動をすると，更に悪くなりますから，控えてください.

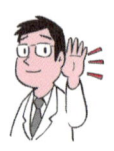

[Listening comprehension]　　　（解答は別冊）

152. What is the most likely diagnosis?
153. What are the doctor's instructions?

Case 23　急性緑内障発作（75歳女性）

Dr. What is the problem?
Pt. My right eye hurts and it gets red. Now I have difficulty seeing.
Dr. When did it start?
Pt. The day before yesterday.
Dr. Why didn't you come to see me earlier?
Pt. Yesterday, I felt ill, so I went to see my doctor.
Dr. Your internal eye pressure, which is over 50mmHg, indicates that you may have glaucoma. Your pain and discomfort is from an acute attack. You need to be treated with eye drops and receive photocoagulation therapy. I've already put some drops in your eye, so we'll have to wait to see how they work.

*****

Dr. Fortunately, the drops seem to have worked well, and the pressure has gone down. I'll perform iris photocoagulation therapy to prevent another attack.
Pt. I can see much better now.

Dr. どうしましたか．
Pt. 右の目が痛いし，赤くなり，見えにくいのです．
Dr. いつからですか．
Pt. 一昨日からです．
Dr. なぜもっと早く来なかったの．
Pt. 昨日は，気分が悪く，内科に行きました．
Dr. 眼圧の値，50mmHg以上ありますが，それからすると緑内障でしょう．緑内障の発作で痛くて気分が悪かったのでしょう．点眼薬での治療と，光凝固治療が必要です．もうすでにお薬を点眼しましたので，目薬の効果を見ますから，しばらく待っていてください．

*****

Dr. 縮瞳薬が効いて，眼圧が正常に下がったようです．良かったですね．緑内障発作が二度と起こらないように，虹彩の光凝固手術をしておきましょう．
Pt. 見えやすくなりました．

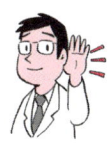

[Listening comprehension]　　（解答は別冊）

154. What is the most likely diagnosis?
155. What was the next step, after applying myotic drops?

PART 2

Basic Medical Writing 編

- 基本編　　138
- 応用編　　143

A 基本的な Writing Patterns を紹介します.

■ ～を訴えて来院（入院）する

> **A 37-year-old man visits my clinic** + **complaining of a high fever.**
> 37歳男性が，高熱を訴えてクリニックに来院する．

▶ Complaining of の代わりに with を用いることができます．

あてはめましょう！ 次の枠内に下記の用語をあてはめましょう．

(a) A 37-year-old man [a] + complaining of a high fever.
(b) A 37-year-old man visits my clinic + [b] a high fever.

(a) visited my clinic, presented to the office 来院した，was admitted to the hospital 入院した
(b) complaining of 高熱を訴えて，with 高熱を伴い，because of 高熱のために

次の Report を書いてみましょう． （解答は別冊）

1. 47歳男性が慢性的にくりかえす上腹部痛を訴えて来院する．
2. 26歳男性が吐き気，嘔吐，39.5度の高熱および広範に渡る腹部の痛みを訴える．

■ ～という所見がある（ない）

> **There is (no) [(a)所見].**
> There is no tumor in the stomach.　　胃には腫瘍は認められない．

(a) no history of any recent measles contact　はしかの患者との接触歴はない
　　nothing remarkable about it.　それについて特に目立った所見はない

次の Report を書いてみましょう． （解答は別冊）

3. マンモグラフィーで異常（abnormalities）は認められない．

■ 症状に随伴症状がある

> 症状 is present with 随伴症状 .
> Headache is present with nausea. 吐き気を伴う頭痛がある.

次の Report を書いてみましょう. （解答は別冊）

4. 目の痛みを伴い，緑内障が認められる.
5. 吐き気と嘔吐がある.（nausea and vomiting）
6. 軟部組織に腫脹がある.（soft tissue swelling）

> ◆ "present" を次の単語に置き換えることができます.
> 所見 is present
> is found.   が認められる.
> is observed. が認められる.
> is seen   が認められる.
> is detected が認められる. 症状を発見する.
> is noted   が認められる（指摘される）.
> 参照：医系文では受身形が多いが，日本語へ翻訳する時は能動態で訳す方が自然な場合も多い.

次の Report を書いてみましょう. （解答は別冊）

7. 10 mm の腫瘤が，マンモグラフィーによるスクリーニング検査で認められた.
8. 腹痛ならびに帯下の減少が認められた.
9. 吐き気を伴う頭痛が認められる.

■ 他の表現

> The abdomen is solid/tender to palpation.　腹部は触診で固い.
> The size of the mass measures A cm to palpation.　腫瘤は触診で A cm ある.
> The lung is clear to auscultation.　聴診上呼吸音は正常である.
> The skin rash is accompanied by blebs on inspection.　視診で皮疹には水疱がみられる.
> The vital signs are within normal limits.　バイタルサインは正常範囲内である.

次の Report を書いてみましょう. （解答は別冊）

10. ピロリ菌抗体試験は陽性である.
11. 測定で，血圧は 120/74 mmHg. である.
12. 聴診上，呼吸音は正常で，心音は整，心雑音は認めない.

■ 検査の結果，～（症状・病名）であることがわかった

The test shows 症状／病名 .
The radiography shows (a disease/symptoms).
レントゲン検査の結果，（病名 / 症状）があることがわかる．
The values are consistent with disease.
検査の値から，（病名）である（一致する，矛盾はない）．

◆ **Show** を次の単語に置き換えることができます．
The radiography shows a malignant tumor.
　　　　　　　 reveals
　　　　　　　 discloses
　　　　　　　 substantiates（立証する，実証する）
　　　　　　　 demonstrates（立証する，実証する）

次の Report を書いてみましょう． （解答は別冊）

13. 検査値はクレアチン 1.2 mg/dL，アラニン・アミノトランスフェラーゼ 3430 IU/L，アルカリホスファターゼ 352 IU/L およびプロトロビン時間 15 秒で，これらの値はウイルス性肝炎に矛盾しない．
14. 呼吸数は 36/分，血圧は 140/110 mmHg，脈拍は 120/分，血中グルコース値は 140 mg/dl．

■ ～と診断する

The patient was diagnosed with diabetes. 糖尿病と診断された．
Diabetes was diagnosed. 診断は糖尿病であった．
His (most likely) diagnosis is diabetes. 糖尿病である（可能性が最も高い）．

■ ～の治療を受けている

The patient has been treated for diabetes. 糖尿病の治療を受けている．
The patient is being treated with antihypertensive drugs. 降圧剤を用いて治療している．

■ ～の治療として～をする

The treatment involves/is considered surgical care. 治療として外科手術をする．
　　　　　　　　　　　　　　　　　　　　　　conservative therapy 治療として保存療法をする．

A 基本編

次の Report を書いてみましょう. （解答は別冊）

15. この疾患では，高齢の患者には，若い患者と比べ外科手術をあまり行わない．
16. 初期糖尿病の治療で重要な事は，食事療法と運動療法である．

■ 〜の薬剤を服用する（服用を中止する）

> **The patient <u>takes/is given/is administered</u> NSAIDs.** NSAIDs を服用する．
> **has discontinued NSAIDs** NSAIDs の服用を中止する

あてはめましょう！ 次の枠内に下記の用語をあてはめましょう．

(a) A patient receives _____.
(b) A doctor _____ surgery.
(c) A doctor applies _____.
(d) A doctor _____ a patient on Tamiflu.
(e) Tamiflu was _____.
(f) A doctor places a patient on _____.

(a) surgery 手術を受ける，conservative therapy 保存的治療を受ける，IV injection 静脈注射を受ける，IV drop infusion 点滴を受ける
(b) performs, gives, undertakes 施行する
(c) eye drops 目薬をさす，lotion ローションを塗る，topical cream 塗り薬を塗る，ointment 軟膏を塗る
(d) started 投与を始めた
(e) discontinued, stopped 投与を中止した
(f) bed rest 絶対安全とする，gastric lavage 胃洗浄をする

次の Report を書いてみましょう. （解答は別冊）

17. 患者は，潰瘍形成を引き起こす可能性のある非ステロイド消炎鎮痛剤（NSAIDs）は服用していない．
18. 医師は，かぜのような細菌性でない疾患には抗生剤を投与しない．

■ 病気の経過の説明

Diabetes improved. 糖尿病は改善した.
resolved 回復した, subsided 治まった
is persisting 継続している, cured 治癒した, aggravated 悪化した, ameliorated 改善した
Breast cancer returns/comes back/recurs 乳がんが再発する

次のreportを書いてみましょう. （解答は別冊）

19. 痛みが素早く消失した.
20. AとBの薬剤を両方投与した結果，腎機能は改善し，ほとんどの症状は治まった.

■ 指示をする

The doctor advises the patient to have enough rest. 患者に十分に休養するよう指示する.
     instructs

次のreportを書いてみましょう. （解答は別冊）

21. 医師は患者にその感染症のために，一日3回抗生剤を服用するよう指示する.
22. 医師は患者にバランスのとれた食事をとり，日常的に運動を行い，十分な休養をとること，さらに病気の原因となるものを避けることを指示する.

> **研究：case reportの時制**
>
> Case reportは普通現在形で書かれます．しかし，すでに行われた一連の処置について述べているものは過去形を用いています．一般的に患者さんからの情報（話）は過去形を用います．

B Case Report を書いてみましょう.

内　科

CASE 1 　胃潰瘍 stomach ulcer　　　　　　　　　　　　　　　（解答は別冊）

47歳男性，慢性的な腹痛を主訴に来院．痛みは空腹時に悪化し，食後は改善する．喫煙はしない．夕食時に飲酒をする．NSAIDs（非ステロイド系消炎鎮痛剤）は使用していない．ピロリ菌抗体検査は陽性．
指示：飲酒を制限するように指示する．

> 【ヒント】　慢性的な腹痛　chronic abdominal pain
> 　　　　　痛みが悪化する　the pain becomes worse
> 　　　　　ピロリ菌抗体検査　his pyloric antibody test
> 　　　　　飲酒を制限する　limit alcohol consumption

CASE 2-1 　ウイルス性急性肝炎 viral hepatitis　　　　　　　　（解答は別冊）

26歳男性．吐き気，嘔吐，38.5度の熱および広範な腹部の痛みを訴える．熱のために時折，アセトアミノフェンを使用しているがそれ以外の薬は飲んでいない．検査で，血圧は120/74 mmHgである．聴診上，呼吸音は正常で心音整，心雑音を認めず．肝は12 cm 触知し，同部位の圧痛を認める．

> 【ヒント】　広範な腹部の痛み diffuse abdominal pain
> 　　　　　肝は12 cm 触知する the patient's liver measures 12 cm
> 　　　　　圧痛がある is tender to palpation

CASE 2-2 　ウイルス性急性肝炎 viral hepatitis　　　　　　　　（解答は別冊）

検査値はクレアチニン 1.2 mg/dL，アラニン・アミノトランスフェラーゼ 3430 IU/L，アルカリホスファターゼ 352 IU/L およびプロトロンビン時間 15 秒で有意である．これらの値はウイルス性急性肝炎に矛盾しない．
指示：病態の悪化を防ぐために，入院して増悪因子誘因を避け，十分に休養をとるように指示する．

> 【ヒント】　検査値は，〜で有意である laboratory values are significant for 〜

これらの値は，〜(病名)と矛盾しない(一致する) all values are consistent with 〜
〜するように指示する you advise him to 〜
病態の悪化 a worsening of the condition

CASE 3 胃癌 gastric cancer （解答は別冊）

51歳男性．体重減少，下痢及び悪心，嘔吐を主訴に来院．約2週間前からタール便がみられ，ピロリ菌抗体検査は陽性．上部消化管内視鏡検査で胃癌を認めたため，腹部CT及び超音波内視鏡検査が施行された．その結果手術適応と判断し，患者にその旨説明した．

【ヒント】　〜を主訴に来院 presents to your clinic with chief complaints of 〜
　　　　　検査は陽性 test is positive
　　　　　上部消化管内視鏡検査で on upper endoscopic exam

CASE 4 急性胃炎 acute gastritis （解答は別冊）

28歳女性．急性の胃痙攣様の痛みを主訴として来院．悪心と嘔吐を認めるが，吐下血や貧血は認めない．痛みは，食事または市販の制酸剤で軽減する．
指示：患者に消化の良い食事を摂るように，また，制酸剤を服用するように指示する．
予後：食生活の改善と制酸剤の服用で完全に消失した．

【ヒント】　急性の胃痙攣様の痛み acute cramping pain
　　　　　吐下血や貧血 hematemesis, melena or anemia
　　　　　痛みは〜で軽減する the pain is relieved by
　　　　　消化の良い食事を摂る eat easily-digestible food
　　　　　症状は〜で完全に消失した her symptoms resolve completely with 〜
　　　　　予後 prognosis

小児科

CASE 5-1 川崎病 Kawasaki disease （解答は別冊）

1歳男児．高熱にて来院．咽頭発赤とイチゴ舌があり，咽頭A群溶連菌検査は陰性．麻黄湯を処方したが高熱が持続し2日後再受診．四肢末端の掌蹠紅斑と硬性浮腫，頸部リンパ節腫大があり．白血球数 19500/μL, 血小板数 370,000/μL, CRP 6.5 mg/dl であり入院．口唇発赤，全身皮疹も出現し，心エコー検査にて，軽度冠動脈拡張もみられた．

【ヒント】　咽頭発赤とイチゴ舌 pharynx redness and strawberry tongue

高熱が持続する the high-grade fever persists
四肢末端の掌蹠紅斑 redness on the hands and the soles of the feet (erythema of the tip extremities)
硬性浮腫 hard edema
頸部リンパ節腫大 enlarged lymph node
口唇発赤 red lips
全身皮疹 a full body rash
軽度冠動脈拡張 mild coronary vasodilatation(mild coronary dilation)

CASE 5-2　川崎病 Kawasaki disease　　（解答は別冊）

川崎病と診断し，小児用バファリン®とγ-グロブリンを投与し，入院4病日解熱した．血液検査，心エコー検査所見も改善し，入院12病日退院，外来フォローアップとした．

【ヒント】　解熱した the fever is reduced
入院4病日 the fourth day following her admission
外来フォローアップとした is scheduled for regular follow-up

CASE 6-1　気管支喘息 bronchial asthma　　（解答は別冊）

2歳女児．RSV感染症，喘息性気管支炎の既往あり．家族歴で父は気管支喘息．深夜から咳，喘鳴があり早朝来院．呼吸障害，口唇チアノーゼ，呼気性喘鳴があり，心拍数145/分，SPO₂ 88%．気管支喘息発作として，酸素投与下にステロイドの点滴静注を開始，その後ベネトリン®の吸入療法を施行し症状は改善．

【ヒント】　〜（病名）の既往あり has a history of 〜（病名）
口唇チアノーゼ，呼気性喘鳴 lip cyanosis, expiratory wheezes(wheezing)
（A症状）がある A is present
酸素投与下に under oxygen inhalation therapy

CASE 6-2　気管支喘息 bronchial asthma　　（解答は別冊）

母親に気管支喘息治療・管理ガイドラインについて説明し，キュバール®吸入薬，シングレア®，ホクナリンテープ®を処方し2日後発作は消失．RAST検査で，家ダニとハウスダストに強い陽性反応を示したため，生活環境を改善するように指示した．ピークフローメーター，喘息日誌を家族に渡し，継続治療とした．

【ヒント】　Aについて説明する explain A（注意：explainのあとにaboutはつかない）
キュバール®吸入薬 QVAR, シングレア® Singulair, ホクナリンテープ® Hokunalin
発作は消失 the attacks subsided
〜に強い陽性反応を示す demonstrates strong positive reactions to 〜

CASE 7　左外鼠径ヘルニア（嵌頓）left external inguinal hernia（incarcerated） （解答は別冊）

生後5ヵ月男児．夜中に激しく泣いて泣きやまないため急病センターを受診．左鼠径部に圧痛を伴う腫瘤がみられ，鼠径ヘルニア嵌頓と診断された．小児外科医により徒手整復され，2日後全身麻酔下に根治術を受け，術後の経過は良好であった．

【ヒント】　左鼠径部に in the left groin area
　　　　　圧痛を伴う腫瘤 a tender mass
　　　　　徒手整復される a closed reduction（CR）procedure was performed
　　　　　根治術を施行 a radical operation was performed
　　　　　その後の経過は良好であった favorable prognosis reported/Post-operative course was uneventful

CASE 8　突発性発疹 convulsive attack （解答は別冊）

生後6ヵ月男児．39.5度の高熱とけいれん発作があり来院．けいれんは3分間持続し，熱性けいれんを疑い，ダイアップ坐薬挿入，咽頭発赤，大泉門の軽度膨隆がみられたが，頸部硬直なし．白血球 7500/mm^3，CRPは 0.0 mg/dl．熱性けいれんと診断し，ダイアップ坐薬，アルピニー坐薬を処方．3日間高熱が続いたのち解熱した．皮疹が出現し，突発性発疹と診断した．その後けいれん発作はなし．

【ヒント】　〜がある A is present
　　　　　〜がない B is absent
　　　　　大泉門膨隆や頸部硬直 bulging anterior fontanel and cervical rigidity
　　　　　高熱が続きその後解熱する a high-grade fever lasted and then subsided

婦人科

CASE 9　カンジダ腟炎 candidiasis （解答は別冊）

38歳女性．3日前より外陰部掻痒感と帯下あり．帯下は白色・ヨーグルト，あるいはカッテージチーズ状．1週間前に気管支炎で抗生物質内服の既往あり．腟分泌物の検鏡で酵母様真菌をみとめる．抗真菌剤の外用と腟坐薬の挿入を1週間続け，完治となる．

【ヒント】　陰部掻痒感 vulvar itching
　　　　　カッテージチーズ状 cottage cheese-like
　　　　　〜（病名）で抗生物質内服をする takes oral antibiotics for the treatment of 〜
　　　　　腟分泌物の検鏡で on microscopic examination of vaginal discharge
　　　　　〜を続け，完治となる fully recovers following successful treatment with 〜

CASE 10　子宮内膜症 endometriosis　　　(解答は別冊)

32歳女性．6年前より月経困難症が徐々に増悪．月経過多はない．2年前より排便痛と性交痛(深部痛)出現．内診にてダグラス窩に有痛性の硬結．子宮の可動性制限あり．血中CA125：60 U/mlと軽度上昇．Gn-RHアナログによる偽閉経療法を6ヵ月間施行．症状改善が認められ，その後対症療法にてフォローとなる．

【ヒント】　徐々に増悪する has gradually increased in severity
　　　　　内診にて on pelvic examination
　　　　　ダグラス窩に in the area of Douglas pouch
　　　　　可動性制限あり mobility is limited
　　　　　〜(数値)と軽度上昇 is raised slightly to 〜(数値)
　　　　　Gn-RHアナログによる偽閉経療法 GnRH-agonist induced menopausal therapy
　　　　　対症療法にてフォローとなる continuing symptomatic supportive treatments are received

> 📌 参照：
> The level of CA 125 in the blood **has increased** slightly to 60 U/mL.
> 前回の検査以来の変化を表すために "has increased" という文型を使います．比較せずに現状を表す場合は "is raised" または，"is elevated" がよく使われます．

CASE 11　子宮外妊娠 ectopic pregnancy(eccyesis)　　　(解答は別冊)

33歳女性．下腹痛と性器出血を主訴に外来受診．尿妊娠反応陽性．最終月経より妊娠8週4日．エコーにて子宮内に胎嚢なし，ダグラス窩にフリースペースを認め，右卵管腫大あり．腹膜刺激症状陽性にて，婦人科病棟に緊急入院となる．

【ヒント】　最終月経より妊娠8週4日 8 weeks and 4 days pregnant, dated from the first day of her last period
　　　　　〜を認め，胎嚢なし demonstrates 〜, but no gestational sac
　　　　　〜にて(の結果)，婦人科病棟に緊急入院となる is admitted urgently to the gynecology ward as a result of 〜

CASE 12　バルトリン腺膿瘍 Bartholin's abscess　　　(解答は別冊)

34歳女性．3年前からバルトリン腺嚢胞の穿刺の既往あり．5日前より外陰痛と外陰部腫瘤感あり．視診上腟入口部左側に直径3センチの圧痛を伴う柔らかい腫瘤を認める．1%キシロカインにて局所麻酔ののち，メスにて膿瘍を切開・排膿を施行．内容液は黄色・膿性の粘液で，細菌培養を提出した．

【ヒント】　外陰痛と外陰部腫瘤感 external vulvar pain and a self-palpable vulvar mass
　　　　　圧痛を伴う with tenderness
　　　　　腫瘤を認める a soft tissue mass is detected
　　　　　局所麻酔ののち after applying local anesthesia
　　　　　細菌培養を提出した be submitted for bacterial culture

CASE 13　クラミジア子宮頸管炎 Chlamydial Cervicitis　　（解答は別冊）

19歳女性．帯下の増加を主訴に受診．腟鏡診にて子宮腟部の発赤と頸管より多量の漿液性分泌物を認めた．腟分泌物のPCR検査にて，クラミジア陽性．セックスパートナーの初尿の検査にてもクラミジア陽性．パートナーとともにアジスロマイシン1000 mg内服の単回投与を行う．

【ヒント】　腟分泌物のPCR検査にて(によって) via PCR using a discharge specimen
　　　　　初尿の検査 a first-void urine test
　　　　　〜に1000 mg内服の単回投与を行う A single 1000 mg dose of azithromycin is administered to 〜

CASE 14　更年期障害 climacteric disturbance　　（解答は別冊）

50歳女性．1年前より月経不順．半年前より無月経あり．その頃より顔のほてり，のぼせ，発汗，突発的な動悸あり．2ヵ月前より肩こりと頭痛，イライラ感と不規則な不眠出現．市販の漢方薬を飲んでいたが軽快しないため婦人科受診．初診時のホルモン検査にてエストラジール（E2）の低下と卵胞刺激ホルモン（FSH）の上昇を認める．更年期障害の診断にてホルモン補充療法（HRT）をすすめる．

【ヒント】　無月経 amenorrhea
　　　　　顔のほてり，のぼせ facial flushing, hot flash
　　　　　不規則な不眠 erratic insomnia
　　　　　〜を飲んでいたが症状が軽快しない used 〜 with no resolution of her symptoms
　　　　　A値の低下とB値の上昇を認める demonstrated a decline in A level and an increase in B level

整形外科

CASE 15　手根管症候群 carpal tunnel syndrome　（解答は別冊）

25歳女性．妊娠8ヵ月の間に生じた左手部のしびれ感を主訴に来院．正中神経領域に知覚鈍麻があり，夜間睡眠中に増強する．理学所見ではファーレンテスト陽性．手根管症候群のチネルサイン陽性．母指球の萎縮が認められた．これらの事から，手根管症候群と診断した．治療として正中神経ブロックを行い，軽快した．

【ヒント】　妊娠8ヵ月ごろ in the 8th month of pregnancy
　　　　　～(症状)を主訴に来院 visited the office with a chief complaint of ～
　　　　　知覚鈍麻が増強する hypesthesia increases in sensitivity
　　　　　ファーレンテスト Phalen's test
　　　　　手根管上のチネルサイン Tinel's sign on carpal tunnel
　　　　　(症状～)が認められた～ is observed
　　　　　これらの事から(病名～)と診断した considering these factors, ～ was diagnosed
　　　　　手根管症候群 carpal tunnel syndrome
　　　　　治療として～を行った for treatment, ～ was performed

CASE 16　小児弾撥指 trigger finger in children（弾撥指）　（解答は別冊）

1歳5ヵ月，男児．母親と来院．母親が右母指IP関節の伸展障害に気づき来院．他動的に伸展を試みると，スナップを伴い伸展したが，自動的には不可能であった．長母指屈筋腱に一致した腫瘤を認めたが，圧痛は無かった．他動的屈曲伸展による保存的治療にて4ヵ月後に治癒した．

【ヒント】　右母指IP関節の伸展障害 extension injuries of the IP joint of the right thumb
　　　　　スナップを伴い accompanied by a snapping
　　　　　長母指屈筋腱に in the tendon of the extensor hallucis longus muscle
　　　　　他動的屈曲伸展 passive extension

CASE 17　足底腱膜炎 fasciitis（plantar aponeurositis）　（解答は別冊）

40歳男性．起床時および歩き始めの踵部の疼痛を主訴に来院．X線検査にて踵骨棘を認めた．同部の圧痛を認めた．毎日のストレッチを指示し，足底装具を処方した．

【ヒント】　踵部の疼痛 pain in the calcaneal region
　　　　　起床時および歩き始め upon arising in the morning and when starting walking
　　　　　踵骨棘 calcaneal spurs
　　　　　毎日のストレッチ daily stretch exercises
　　　　　足底装具 custom-made arch supports

CASE 18　有痛性外脛骨 painful os tibiale externum　　　(解答は別冊)

10歳男児がスポーツ時の左足内側部の疼痛を主訴に来院．舟状骨結節部に腫脹と圧痛がある．X線検査により舟状骨の内側に副骨を認めた．スポーツ活動の制限を指示．ストレッチ，テーピングの指導，温熱治療を行い数ヵ月の経過で治癒する．再発防止のためのストレッチの重要性を強調した．

【ヒント】　左足内側部の on the inside(inner side)of the left foot
　　　　　舟状骨結節部に on the scaphoid tubercle
　　　　　種子骨 accesssory bone
　　　　　舟状骨の内側に inside the os navicular

皮膚科

CASE 19-1　左胸背部帯状疱疹 left thoracic herpes zoster　　　(解答は別冊)

60歳女性が痛みを伴う発疹を訴えて来院する．痛みは3日前から生じている．痛みは左胸に限局しており，左背部にも放散している．昨日から左胸に赤みを伴う小水疱に気付いている．

【ヒント】　～に限局している is found localized to ～
　　　　　左胸背部に located on the left chest and back
　　　　　～にも放散している with radiation to ～

CASE 19-2　左胸背部帯状疱疹 left thoracic herpes zoster　　　(解答は別冊)

患者は慢性腎不全のため5年前から血液透析を受けている．胸部X線撮影では肋骨に異常を認めない．心電図所見にも異常は認めない．
診断：左胸背部帯状疱疹

【ヒント】　血液透析 hemodialysis
　　　　　慢性腎不全 chronic renal failure
　　　　　肋骨に異常 costal abnormality

CASE 20-1　アレルギー性紫斑病 anaphylactoid purpura　　　(解答は別冊)

26歳男性が3日前から両下腿から足首にかけて多発する紫斑に気付き来院する．発疹の自覚症状(痒み・痛み)はない．両下腿の腫脹と足関節の痛みを訴える．発疹からの皮膚生検にて，真皮上層の小静脈の変性と血管周囲性に赤血球と好中球の浸潤を認める．

【ヒント】　多発する spread over
　　　　　両下腿から足首にかけて a wide area of his lower thighs and ankles
　　　　　自覚症状 subjective symptoms
　　　　　下腿の腫脹 lower thigh bloating
　　　　　小静脈の変性 degeneration of small veins
　　　　　血管周囲性に in the surrounding area of blood vessels
　　　　　赤血球と好中球の浸潤 infiltration of neutrophils and erythrocytes

📌（文の組み立て方）

（1）which を用いて「紫斑」のあとに紫斑の詳しい説明を追加する.
両下腿から足首にかけて多発する紫斑に気付き来院する.

（2）真皮上層の小静脈の変性 / と血管周囲性に / 赤血球と好中球の浸潤 / を認める.
部位を表す箇所は，前置詞（in や on）などのフレーズにして，それぞれ「真皮上層の」は「小静脈の変性」のあとに，「血管周囲性に」は「赤血球と好中球の浸潤」のあとにつけ足します.
"degeneration of small veins in the upper dermis and infiltration of neutrophils and erythrocytes in the surrounding area of blood vessels."が目的語となります.
この目的語は，主語・述語（皮膚生検にて認めた→皮膚生検が認めた Skin biopsy reveals）のあとに置きます.

CASE 20-2　アレルギー性紫斑病 anaphylactoid purpura　（解答は別冊）

尿検査では潜血反応を認める．1 週間前から感冒様症状があり，発熱はないが，のどの痛みを感じている．患者に腎炎の可能性があることを伝え，入院して精査するように指示する．
診断：両下腿アナフラクトイド紫斑および紫斑性腎炎の疑い.

【ヒント】　潜血反応 the occult blood test
　　　　　感冒様症状 cold-like symptoms
　　　　　入院して精査する needs to be hospitalized for further examination
　　　　　アナフラクトイド紫斑 anaphylactoid purpura

CASE 21-1　悪性黒色腫 malignant melanoma：皮膚生検　（解答は別冊）

51 歳男性が右足底の色素斑を訴えて来院する．色素斑は最近隆起してきて，時に出血がみられる．視診と触診では悪性黒色腫が疑われる．感染（化膿）はしていない.

【ヒント】　色素斑 pigmented patches
　　　　　右足底の（にある）in the right plantar region
　　　　　視診と触診では on visual inspection and palpation
　　　　　悪性黒色腫 malignant melanoma

CASE 21-2　悪性黒色腫 malignant melanoma：皮膚生検 　　　　　　　　（解答は別冊）

キシロカインの局所麻酔下に色素斑を全摘出し，病理組織診断を行う．その結果，異型の色素細胞の増殖を認め，診断が確定する．入院の上，画像診断による転移巣の検索を行う．

【ヒント】　全摘出し are fully removed
　　　　　局所麻酔下 under local anesthesia
　　　　　病理組織診断 a histopathologic diagnosis
　　　　　異型の色素細胞の増殖 atypical pigmentary cell growth
　　　　　画像診断 diagnostic imaging

CASE 22-1　皮脂欠乏性湿疹 asteatotic eczema 　　　　　　　　（解答は別冊）

70歳男性が両下肢のかゆみを訴える．両下肢全体に乾燥と鱗屑がみられ，多数の掻破痕がみられる．鱗屑からの真菌検査は陰性である．乾皮症の既往歴はない．

【ヒント】　両下肢 under both lower thighs
　　　　　乾燥と鱗屑 dryness and dander
　　　　　破痕掻 scratch scars
　　　　　〜がみられる　〜 are observed
　　　　　真菌検査 fungal tests
　　　　　乾皮症 asteatotic eczema

CASE 22-2　皮脂欠乏性湿疹 asteatotic eczema 　　　　　　　　（解答は別冊）

診断：両下肢皮脂欠乏性湿疹（皮脂欠乏性皮膚炎または乾皮症）．
治療：1日1回，入浴後に，保湿剤と弱いステロイド（副腎皮質ホルモン）軟膏を塗布するように指示する．生活指導：患者に石鹸の使用をひかえさせる．
経過：患者の症状は2週間でほぼ消失する．

【ヒント】　保湿剤と弱いステロイド（副腎皮質ホルモン）軟膏 a moisturizer and weak steroidal
　　　　　　ointments(topical corticosteroid)
　　　　　入浴後 after bathing
　　　　　ほぼ消失する have mainly subsided

眼　科

CASE 23　近視 myopia　　　　　　　　　　　　　　　　　　　　　　（解答は別冊）

12歳男児．半年前から，学校で，黒板の字がかすんで見えにくいと訴える．視力：RV = 0.4 (1.0x − 1.5D)．LV = 0.3 (1.0x − 1.75D)．屈折検査にて両眼ともに− 2.0Dの近視を認めた．両眼ともに− 1.25Dの眼鏡処方をした．両眼にて矯正視力＝(1.2)．

　【ヒント】　屈折検査 refraction test

CASE 24　弱視 amblyopia　　　　　　　　　　　　　　　　　　　　　（解答は別冊）

4歳女児．左眼が見えにくそうなことに母親が気付く．視力：RV = 1.0，LV = 0.2 (0.5x + 3.0D)．左眼の近部視力 = 0.5．弱視と診断．左眼に眼鏡処方し，健眼の右眼にアイパッチにてペナリゼーションをし，経過観察中．半年後の現在，左眼の弱視は徐々に改善中．

　【ヒント】　左眼が見えにくい has difficulty with vision in her left eye
　　　　　　弱視 amblyopia
　　　　　　経過観察中 has been followed up
　　　　　　参照：遠視性弱視 hyperopic astigmatism，矯正視力 correcting visual acuity，
　　　　　　近方視力・近見視力 near visual acuity，片眼視力 unilateral visual acuity

CASE 25　急性結膜浮腫　acute conjunctival chemosis　　　　　　　　　（解答は別冊）

5歳女児．急に夜中に白目が腫れて，眼を閉じても腫れた部分の白目がとびだしている．救急車にて来院．聞くと，お隣のネコをさわった後に腫れたとのこと．消炎剤の点眼薬と抗生剤の点眼薬を処方．翌日には治癒．救急車の利用法も考慮されたい．

　【ヒント】　白目の腫れ abrupt chemosis, swelling of the conjunctiva (the white part of the eyes)
　　　　　　ネコをさわる stroking a cat
　　　　　　消炎剤の点眼薬と抗生剤の点眼薬 antibiotic drops and anti-phlogistic drops

CASE 26　眼底出血 hemophthalmia/ocular hemorrhage　　　　　　　　（解答は別冊）

45歳女性．約10年前から糖尿病があり，内科にて治療中．1週間前から視力低下あり．前眼部には異常なく，眼底に無数の出血斑，白斑，浮腫を認める．網膜の中心の黄斑部に出血が及んだために視力低下を生じた．もっと早期から眼底のチェックが望まれた．網膜の光凝

固治療により，視力維持に努めたい．

【ヒント】　視力低下 a decline in visual acuity
　　　　　無数の出血斑，白斑，浮腫 numerous blood spots (hemorrhagic macule), leukoderma, and edema
　　　　　黄斑部に出血 macular bleeding
　　　　　網膜の光凝固治療 photocoagulation of the retina

CASE 27　ぶどう膜炎（虹彩毛様体脈絡膜炎）uveitis (anterior uveitis, iridocyclitis) (解答は別冊)

25歳男性．2週間前からクモの巣のようなモノが見え，3日前から白目が充血．眼の痛みも生じて来た．視力も低下，毛様充血様充血が強く，前房の混濁は強度．
ステロイドの結膜下注射および点眼薬，消炎剤の内服により，やや改善．今後も治療が必要である．
指示：アルコール摂取を制限するよう指示する．

【ヒント】　クモの巣のようなモノが見えること spider web-like visual spots
　　　　　白目が充血 hyperemia in the white part of the eyes
　　　　　視力が低下 visual acuity has deteriorated
　　　　　前房の混濁 opacity in the anterior chamber
　　　　　消炎剤の内服および点眼薬，ステロイドの注射 the oral administration of antiphlogistic, steroid drops, and steroid injection

▶参考文献

1. Phillip Brottman, MD., Sonia Reichert, MD.: USMLE ^{TM} Step 2 CS : COMPLEX CASES. KAPLAN Publishing, New York, 2007
2. Eugene C. Toy MD., John T. Patran, Jr. MD., Fabrizia, Faustinella, MD. PHD., S. Elizabeth Cruse, MD.: Case Files Internal Medicine. The Mc-Graw Hill, 2007
3. Medicine 1, 2, 3. Collier MacMillan International, 1969
4. マリア・ジョルフィ, J. パトリック・バロン: English for Doctors. メジカルビュー社, 2007
5. 辻谷真一郎: メディカプラス 2000（1 〜 12）. トライアリスト, 2000
6. Michael Agnes: Webster's New World Dictionary. Wiley Publishing, 2003
7. David Burke: BiZ Talk1,2,3. Optima Books, 1998

医学英語 Communication & Writing 能力アップ！

2012 年 4 月 1 日　第 1 版第 1 刷発行
2013 年 4 月 15 日　第 1 版第 2 刷発行

著　者	土居　治　　DOI, Osamu
	西村真澄　　NISHIMURA, Masumi
	David Chart
発行者	市井輝和
発行所	株式会社金芳堂
	〒 606-8425 京都市左京区鹿ケ谷西寺ノ前町 34 番地
	振替　01030-1-15605
	電話　075-751-1111（代）
	http://www.kinpodo-pub.co.jp/
印　刷	亜細亜印刷株式会社
製　本	有限会社清水製本所

© 土居　治，西村真澄，David Chart，2012
落丁・乱丁本は直接小社へお送りください．お取替え致します．

Printed in Japan
ISBN978-4-7653-1519-7

JCOPY ＜(社)出版者著作権管理機構　委託出版物＞

本書の無断複写は著作権法上での例外を除き禁じられています．複写される場合は，そのつど事前に，(社)出版者著作権管理機構（電話 03-3513-6969，FAX 03-3513-6979，e-mail: info@jcopy.or.jp）の許諾を得てください．

●本書のコピー，スキャン，デジタル化等の無断複製は著作権法上での例外を除き禁じられています．本書を代行業者等の第三者に依頼してスキャンやデジタル化することは，たとえ個人や家庭内の利用でも著作権法違反です．

医学英語 Communication & Writing 能力アップ！

解答編

Part 1　Communication 編

1. Do you have chest pain when coughing?
2. Do you have foot pain when climbing stairs?
3. Do you have shortness of breath when lying down?
4. Are you short of breath during strenuous activity?
5. Do you hear any wheezing when breathing?
6. Do you get dizzy with exertion?
7. Do you get dizzy when not eating for a period of time?
8. Do you feel lightheaded when dizzy?
9. Have you ever been told you have rheumatic fever?
10. Have you ever had thyroid problems?
11. Have you ever lost consciousness or your balance upon standing?
12. Have you ever been awoken from sleep due to coughing?
13. Have you ever had chest pressure or an irregular heartbeat?
14. Have you ever had a cardiac catheterization or heart surgery?
15. Have you ever noticed yourself wheezing?
16. Have there been any changes in your health?
17. When did you experience this pain last?
18. When did you feel this pain?
19. When did you get this pain?
20. When did you first notice blood in your urine?
21. Do you feel a swimming sensation in your head?
22. Do you feel inbalanced?
23. What makes the swelling go down?
24. What do you think causes your abdominal pain, for example as eating raw foods, like meat, eggs, and fish, or international travel?
25. Would you please describe your chest pain? For example, pressure-like or heavy?
26. Is it worse in the morning or evening?
27. Does the pain occur at rest or with exertion, stress, after eating or moving your arms?
28. Do you know of any possible causes for your dizziness?
29. stomachache

30. C
31. Please lie face up with your knees bent.
32. Please lie face down.
33. Please loosen your belt and lower your pants.
34. Please lie down here on your back, with your head at this end.
35. Please lie on your left side.
36. B
37. Does the pain radiate to your lower back?
38. Does the rash spread to other parts of your body?
39. Does it hurt when I push here and release?
40. Does the pain occur suddenly or gradually?
41. Is your dizziness constant or does it occur intermittently?
42. Do you have diarrhea? How many bowel movements do you have a day?
43. When does dizziness first occur?
44. Have you noticed anything that precipitates an attack?
45. Does anything make the pain better or worse?
46. chest pain
47. It is in the middle and across the left side of the chest.
48. angina
49. The test reveals no specific abnormalities.
50. You can take a rapid HIV test and a rapid HAV test.
51. Rapid diagnostic flu tests are best used within the first 48 hours after symptoms appear to decide whether or not antiviral drugs are used.
52. We can get the results in 10 minutes.
53. You need to be admitted to the hospital.
54. You need to stay overnight in the hospital for an operation.
55. I think you are most likely experiencing a heart attack (myocardial infarction).
56. We'll need to do an X-ray to see if you have pneumonia.
57. After assessing these tests, I'll decide whether or not you should have surgical treatment.
58. The test gives us some idea of whether the mass is solid or cystic.
59. The risk of stroke as a result of this operation is lower than the risk of a stroke if nothing is done.
60. You need to stay in the hospital for observation for 4 to 6 hours.
61. You'll feel a sharp prick.
62. The results of the medical check-up.
63. A, D
64. gingivitis (inflammation around the wisdom tooth) and dental caries.
65. Please drink enough fluids.
66. Please take moderate exercise.
67. Please take your medications as instructed
68. Please take one capsule orally.
69. Please apply topical cream a poultice ointment, as needed.
70. Please take two tablets orally, three times a day for 7 days.
71. You need to make an appointment for the second visit now.
72. hypertension
73. Did you notice if the pain goes away?
74. Did you notice when it started?
75. Did you notice when it hurts, gets better, or gets worse?
76. Did you notice if the pain comes and goes?
77. Did you notice if the pain is constant or intermittent?
78. Have you noticed your child has blood in his stool?
79. When did you notice your child had hearing difficulties?
80. Does your daughter have three days of fever?
81. Does he have any other symptoms, outside of diarrhea?
82. Does your child have a barking cough when breathing?
83. Is the coughing accompanied by difficulty breathing?
84. Is the abdominal pain accompanied by nausea, vomiting, diarrhea or constipation?
85. Is the seizure accompanied by high fever and a disturbance of consciousness?
86. vomiting
87. intussusception
88. Please come back here in a week to see if he can return to school?
89. If your son is short of breath at night, please use this inhaled drug as needed. If the situation doesn't change for the better, please take him to an emergency room ASAP. (as soon as possible).
90. If a seizure lasts longer than 10 to 15 minutes, please take him immediately to the hospital.
91. T
92. F
93. Does your child drink a lot of milk?
94. The bond between mother and child may develop with breast feeding, and it is therefore important that you continue to breastfeed.

95. Please return at the 10 month check up to determine proper growth and development.
96. Did you breastfeed or formula feed?
97. How many times a day does your baby eat weaning food?
98. B, C
99. Because, despite high fever, other abnormalities are not present.
100. urinary tract infection.
101. Can he follow a toy with his eyes?
102. Does he face where sound comes from?
103. Can he speak in two-word sentences?
104. Can he speak words such as mama or dad?
105. Is he able to grasp a toy?
106. Can he use a straw when drinking water?
107. Does he play in a similar manner to his friends?
108. Is your baby getting routine check ups?
109. C
110. B
111. Because he mainly complains of swelling over the right parotid area. And both diseases are conditions that cause swelling over the parotid glands.
112. mumps
113. Have you noticed any swelling in your abdomen?
114. Do you have any discomfort during or after urination or defecation?
115. urine pregnancy test
116. functional uterine bleeding
117. pain in the lower right abdomen
118. B
119. I am going to perform a CT scan to verify the presence of any metastatic disease.
120. Please let me know if you feel any discomfort during the examination.
121. right ovarian cysts
122. Perform presurgery tests including MRI
123. a lot of vaginal discharge
124. Is it painful when you turn over in bed?
125. Is it painful when you start walking?
126. Is it painful when you stand up or sit down?
127. Is it painful when you go up stairs?
128. Is it painful all between your hip and thigh?
129. Does the pain get worse when you bend over?
130. Does the swelling get worse when you walk around?
131. C
132. lumbar disc hernia
133. No, he doesn't.
134. C
135. F
136. T
137. carpal tunnel syndrome
138. nerve conduction test
139. B
140. drug rash
141. discontinue the suspected drug
142. A, C
143. atopic dermatitis
144. take the prescribed drugs and avoid spicy food and alcohol.
145. If your eyes feel dry, gritty or sandy, you may well have dry eyes.
146. Do you sometimes have blurred or double vision? Does your eyes water a lot?
147. If you have double vision, is it when looking with one or two eyes?
148. horudeolum (inflammation of the left eyelid)
149. oral antibiotics, antibiotic eye drops, oral anti-inflammatory drugs, and anti-inflammatory eye drops
150. a foreign object in the left eye
151. The treatment includes using oral antibiotics and anti-inflammatory drugs as well as antibiotic eye drops and anti-inflammatory eye drops.
152. detached retina (RD)
153. go to the hospital for surgery.
154. acute glaucoma attack
155. photocoagulation therapy

Part 2　Basic Medical Writing 編

A

1. A 47-year-old man presents at my clinic complaining of chronic and recurrent upper abdominal pain.
2. A 26-year-old man complains of nausea, vomiting, high fever of 39.5 degrees Centigrade and diffuse abdominal pain.
3. There are no abnormalities on the mammogram.
4. Glaucoma presents with an ocular ache.
5. Nausea and vomiting are present.
6. Soft tissue swelling is present.
7. A 10 mm mass was observed on screening mammography.
8. A decrease in abdominal pain and vaginal discharge was observed.
9. Headache has developed associated with nausea.
10. Pyloric antibody test is positive.
11. On examination, his blood pressure is 120/74 mmHg.
12. The lung is clear to auscultation and the heart is regular without murmurs.
13. Laboratory values are a creatinine of 1.2 mg/dl, alanine aminotransferase (ALT) 3430 IU/L, alkaline phosphatase 352 IU/L and prothrombin time of 15 seconds all of which are consistent with viral hepatitis.
    (Laboratory values: creatine 1.2 mg/dl, alanine aminotransferase (ALT) 3430 IU/L, alkaline phosphatase 352 IU/L and prothrombin time of 15 seconds).
14. The respiratory rate was 36 breaths per minute, the blood pressure 140/110 mmHg, and the pulse 120 beats per minute. The blood glucose level was 140.
15. Elderly patients with this disease are less likely to undergo surgery than younger patients.
16. The important treatment for early stage of diabetes includes dietary therapy as well as exercise therapy.
17. The patient does not take any NSAIDs drugs which might cause ulcer formation.
18. A doctor won't give you an antibiotic for an illness like a cold that isn't likely to be bacterial.
19. The pain subsided quickly.
20. After the combined administration of A and B, renal function improved and most of the symptoms subsided.
21. A doctor instructs the patient to take antibiotics 3 times daily for the infection.
22. A doctor instructs the patient to have a balanced diet, regular exercise, and adequate rest, and to avoid the cause of the disease.

B

Case 1-1

A 47-year-old man presents to your office complaining of chronic abdominal pain. The pain becomes worse when the stomach is empty, and it is relieved after meals. He does not smoke, but drinks alcohol during dinner. He does not take any NSAIDs. His pyloric antibody test is positive.
Instructions: You instruct the patient to limit alcohol consumption.

Case 2-1

A 26-year-old man complains of nausea, vomiting, a fever of 38.5 degrees, and diffuse abdominal pain. He takes no medication except the occasional acetaminophen for fever.
On examination, his blood pressure is 120/74 mmHg. His chest is clear to auscultation and his heart is regular without murmurs. On percussion, the patient's liver measures 12 cm, and is tender to palpation.

Case 2-2

Laboratory values are significant for a creatinine 1.2 mg/dl, alanine animotransferase (ALT) 3430 IU/L, alkaline phosphatase 352 IU/L and prothrombin time of 15 seconds. All values are consistent with viral hepatitis.
Instructions: You recommend hospitalization to prevent a worsening of the condition. You also advice him to get enough rest and avoid all potential disease triggers during hospital stay.

Case 3

A 51-year-old man presents to your clinic with chief complaints of weight loss, diarrhea, nausea, and vomiting. Tarry stool has been observed over the prior two weeks. His H. pyloric antibody test is positive. On upper endoscopic exam, cancer is seen in the region of the stomach. A CT scan and endoscopic ultrasound are then performed. You advise him to have a surgical operation.

Case 4

A 28-year-old woman complains of acute cramping stomach ache. She also has nausea and vomiting. There is no reported hematemesis, melena or anemia. The pain is relieved by food and over-the-counter antacids.
Instructions: You advise the patient to eat easily-digestible food and begin an antacid regimen.
Prognosis: Her symptoms resolve completely with the diet changes and daily medication use.

Case 5-1

A one-year-old boy presents with a high-grade fever. Pharynx redness and strawberry tongue are present. The results of GABHS (Group A Beta-Hemolytic Streptococcus) test are negative. A Kampo called Maoto is administered, but the high-grade fever persists. Two days later, the patient returns.
Redness on the hands and on the soles of the feet (erythema of (palms and soles at) the tip extremities), hard edema, and enlarged neck lymph nodes are present.
The white blood cell count [WBC count] is $19500/\mu l$, platelet count $370,000/\mu l$, and CRP 6.5 mg/dl. The patient is hospitalized, during which time the patient develops red lips and a full body rash. A cardiac ECHO (an echocardiogram) shows mild coronary vasodilatation (mild coronary dilation).

Case 5-2

He is diagnosed with Kawasaki disease. Children's Bufferin and γ globulin is administered. The fever is reduced by the fourth day following his admission. The findings of the blood tests and echocardiography (ECG) likewise improve and the patient is discharged on the 12th day after admission. He is scheduled for regular follow-up.

Case 6-1

A two-year-old girl has a history of RSV infection and asthmatic bronchitis. Her father has a history of bronchial asthma.
She has developed a cough and wheezing since the prior evening, and was brought to my clinic early this morning.
Breathing disorder, lip cyanosis, and expiratory wheezes (wheezing) are present. Heart beat is 145 per minute, and SPO_2 is 88%.
The administration of intravenous steroids was started under oxygen inhalation therapy. Following Venetlin inhalation, symptoms improved.

Case 6-2

I explained to her mother the guidelines for the treatment and management of bronchial asthma. I prescribed QVAR, Singulair® and Hokunalin®.
Two days following treatment, the attacks subsided.
The patient demonstrates strong positive reactions to house mites and dust as reflected in RAST tests. She was therefore counseled to make lifestyle changes.
A peak flow meter and an asthma diary were provided. The patient will require continuous treatment.

Case 7

A 5-month-old boy was taken to the Emergency Department due to incessant crying.
A tender mass was present in the left groin area and the patient was diagnosed with an incarcerated inguinal hernia.
A closed reduction (CR) procedure was performed by a pediatric surgeon. Two days later, the radical operation was performed under general anesthesia. Favorable prognosis was reported (The prognosis has thus been favorable).

Case 8

A 6-month-old boy is brought to the clinic with a high-grade fever of 39.5 and a convulsive seizure. The seizure lasts for 3 minutes. Therefore febrile convulsion is suspected. Then, Diapp is administered. Redness of the pharynx and a slight bulging of the anterior fontanel are present (observed), but cervical rigidity is absent. WBC 7500, CRP 0.0. After a diagnosis of febrile convulsion, Diapp and Alpiny suppositories are prescribed.

A high-grade fever lasted for three days and then subsided. Rashes developed soon after, and the patient was diagnosed with exanthem subitum (roseola infantum). The patient has been seizure-free since treatment.

Case 9

A 38-year-old woman had been suffering from vulvar itching and vaginal discharge for the prior three days. The discharge is described as white and cottage cheese-like. She takes oral antibiotics for the treatment of bronchitis, which she began one week prior to the visit. Yeast-like fungi are identified on microscopic examination of vaginal discharge. She fully recovers following successful treatment with an external application of an anti-fungal agent and the insertion of a vaginal suppository for one week.

Case 10

A 32-year-old woman. Dysmenorrhea has gradually increased in severity over the prior 6 years. There is no hypermenorrhea. She has been suffering from defecation pain and pain with intercourse for the prior two years.
On pelvic examination, a painful mass is found in the area of Douglas' pouch. Uterine mobility is limited. The level of CA125 in the blood is raised slightly to 60 U/ml.
GnRH-agonist induced menopausal therapy is administered for a 6 month duration. The patient's symptoms soon improve. Continuing symptomatic supportive treatments are received.

Case 11

A 33-year-old woman visited my clinic complaining of lower abdominal pain and vaginal bleeding. A urine pregnancy test is positive. She is 8 weeks and 4 days pregnant, dated from the first day of her last period.
Echo demonstrates free space in Douglas' poach, but no gestational sac within the uterus. A large fallopian tube tumor is detected. She is admitted urgently to the gynecology ward as a result of a positive peritoneal irritation sign on examination.

Case 12

A 34-year-old woman with a history of a Bartholin's cysc and a centesis performed three years prior. She has been suffering from external vulvar pain and a self-palpable vulvar mass for the prior 5 days.
A soft tissue mass, 3cm in diameter, with tenderness, is detected on the left vaginal wall upon inspection. After applying local anesthesia (1% xylocaine), an abscess incision is performed with a knife with drainage. The fluid contents are sticky, yellow, and mucus-like. They are submitted for bacterial culture.

Case 13

A 19-year-old female visits the clinic with a chief complaint of increasing vaginal discharge. On speculum examination, redness of the vaginal-cervix region with accompanying serous discharge is observed.
She tests positive for Chlamydia via PCR using a discharge specimen. The first-void urine test for Chlamydia is positive in her sex partner as well. A single 1000 mg dose of azithromycin is administered to both the patient and her partner.

Case 14

A 50-year-old woman presents with menstrual irregularities over the prior year and amenorrhea for the last 6 months. Since then, the patient has experienced facial flashing, hot flashes, sweats, and sudden audible heart beats.
Over the past two months, the patient has experienced a stiff shoulder, headache, irritability, and erratic insomnia. She used over-the counter Kampo, with no resolution of her symptoms.
She then visited a gynecologist, who demonstrated a decline in the patient's estradiol (E2) level and an increase in the follicle-stimulating hormone (FSH) level. The patient is diagnosed with menopause and treated with hormone replacement therapy (HRT).

Case 15

A 25-year-old female visited the office with a chief complaint of left hand numbness, which occurred during the 8th month of pregnancy. Hypesthesia is present in the region of the median nerve, and increases in sensitivity during sleep.
Physiological findings show Phalen's test is positive. Tinel's sign on carpal tunnel is positive. Thenar atrophy is observed. Considering these factors, carpal tunnel syndrome was diagnosed. For treatment, a median nerve block was performed and symptoms improved.

Case 16

A one-year-and-5-month-old (seventeen-month-old) boy presents with his mother. She noticed that her son had extension injuries of the IP joint of the right thumb and brought him to the clinic. The IP joint can be passively extended, accompanied by a snapping. However, the joint cannot be actively extended. A mass located in the tendon of the extensor hallucis longus muscle was observed. but there was no tenderness. 4 months after conservative therapy, involving passive extension and bending exercises, symptoms resolved.

Case 17

A 40-year-old male visited my office with a chief complaint of pain in the calcaneal region, which occurs upon arising in the morning and when starting walking. X-ray shows calcaneal spurs. Tenderness was also present in the same region. Daily stretch exercises were recommended. I prescribed custom-made arch supports.

Case 18

A 10-year-old boy visited my office with a chief complaint of pain on the inside (inner side) of the left foot which occurred during exercise. Swelling and tenderness on the scaphoid tubercle are present. X-ray shows an accessory bone located inside the os navicular. I instruct him to limit athletic activities. Stretching exercises and taping the foot were recommended. Thermal therapy was performed and the condition resolved over a few months. The doctor emphasizes the importance of stretching exercises in prevention of a recurrence.

Case 19-1

A 60 year-old female visited my clinic complaining of a rash accompanied by pain. The pain developed three days ago. The pain is found localized to her left chest and back with radiation to left back region. The patient notes having red blisters yesterday.

Case 19-2

She has been receiving hemodialysis for the last five years to treat chronic renal failure. Chest X-ray shows no costal abnormality. ECG shows no abnormality.
Diagnosis: Herpes zoster (HZ) located on the left chest and back.

Case 20-1

A 26-year-old male presents with widespread purpura, which has spread over a wide area of his lower thighs and ankles. There are no subjective symptoms of itchiness or pain reported. The patient complains of lower thigh bloating and ankle pain.
Skin biopsy reveals degeneration of small veins in the upper dermis and infiltration of neutrophils and erythrocytes in the surrounding area of blood vessels.

Case 20-2

On urine test, the occult blood test was positive. He has been having cold-like symptoms for one week. He has a sore throat, but no fever. The doctor told the patient that he may have nephritis and indicates that he needs to be hospitalized for further examination.
Diagnosis: Suspected anaphylactoid purpura in both lower thighs and purpura nephritis.

Case 21-1

A 51-year-old male visited my clinic complaining of pigmented patches in the right plantar region. The pigmented patches have become more raised recently and are sometimes accompanied by bleeding. On visual inspection and palpation, malignant melanoma is suspected. There is no evidence of infection.

Case 21-2

The pigmented patches are fully removed under local anesthesia with xylocaine and a histopathologic diagnosis is made. Atypical pigmentary cell growth is confirmed. A metastatic focus is checked through diagnostic imaging on admission.

Case 22-1

A 70-year-old male complains of itching under both lower thighs. Dryness and dander as well as many scratch scars are observed over both lower thighs.
Fungal tests are negative. The patient has no history of asteatotic eczema.

Case 22-2

Diagnosis: Asteatotic eczema on under both lower thighs.

Treatment: The patient is instructed to apply a moisturizer and weak steroidal ointments (topical corticosteroid) once a day after bathing.
Instructions: I instruct the patient to refrain from using soap.
Course: Symptoms have mainly subsided over the follow two weeks.

Case 23

A 12-year-old boy complains that he cannot clearly see writing on the blackboard in school over the prior six months.
Visual acuity: RV = 0.4 (1.0x − 1.5D).
　　　　　　　LV = 0.3 (1.0x − 1.75D).
The refraction test shows that he is nearsighted (myopia), (−2.0D). I prescribe glasses of −1.25D (each eye). Corrective vision was 1.2 in both eyes.

Case 24

A mother noticed that her 4-year-old daughter has difficulty with vision in her left eye.
Visual acuity: RV = 1.0, LV = 0.2 (0.5x + 3.0D)
Near visual acuity is 0.5 in the left eye. She was diagnosed with amblyopia.
I prescribed an eyeglass for her left eye and an eye patch over the right eye. She has been followed up. The amblyopia in her left eye is gradually improving as of today, six months after her initial visit.

Case 25

A 5-year-old girl developed swelling of the white part of the eyes. Even when the eyes are closed, folds of edematous conjunctiva are seen to protrude. The patient was transported by ambulance. When being asked about her condition, she mentions that she developed swelling soon after stroking her neighbor's cat. Antibiotic drops and anti-phlogistic drops are prescribed. The eye healed by the following day. An ambulance should be called only in case of emergency.

Case 26

A 45-year-old female has been suffering from diabetes for the past ten years. She has been treated by her physician. There has been a decline in visual acuity during the last week prior to presentation.
There are no abnormalities in the anterior eye. Numerous blood spots (hemorrhagic macule), leukoderma, and edema in the fundus are seen. Visual acuity is compromised due to macular bleeding. Funduscopic examination should have been performed earlier.
〔参照：「～すべきだったのに」と後悔を表す時は，should have been+動詞の過去分詞形 (performed)〕
Photocoagulation of the retina is scheduled in an attempt to maintain visual acuity. (We schedule photocoagulation of the retina in an attempt to salvage visual acuity).

Case 27

A 25-year-old male presents with spider web-like visual spots over the prior two weeks. The patient also developed hyperemia in the white part of the eyes beginning three days ago. Eye pain is also reported. Visual acuity has deteriorated. Strong reticular inflammation is present and opacity in the anterior chamber is apparent.
The patient's condition improves mildly with the oral administration of antiphlogistic, steroid drops, and steroid injection under the conjunctiva. Continuous treatment is recommended.
Instructions: I instruct the patient to limit alcohol consumption.